Small Animal ECGs
An introductory guide

Small Animal ECGs
An introductory guide

Mike Martin

b

**Blackwell
Science**

Copyright © 2000 by

Blackwell Science Ltd

Editorial Offices:
Osney Mead, Oxford OX2 0EL
25 John Street, London WC1N 2BL
23 Ainslie Place, Edinburgh EH3 6AJ
350 Main Street, Malden, MA 02148 5018, USA
54 University Street, Carlton, Victoria 3053, Australia
10, rue Casimir Delavigne, 75006 Paris, France

Other Editorial Offices:

Blackwell Wissenschafts-Verlag GmbH
Kunfürstendamm 57
10707 Berlin, Germany

Blackwell Science KK
MG Kodenmacho Building
7–10 Kodenmacho Nihombashi
Chuo-ku, Tokyo 104, Japan

First published 2000

Produced and typeset in Minion by Gray Publishing,
Tunbridge Wells, Kent
Printed and bound in Great Britain by MPG Books Ltd,
Bodmin, Cornwall

The Blackwell Science logo is a trade mark of Blackwell Science Ltd, registered at the United Kingdom Trade Marks Registry

DISTRIBUTORS
Marston Book Services Ltd
PO Box 269
Abingdon
Oxon OX14 4YN
(*Orders:*   Tel: 01865 206206
                Fax: 01865 721205

USA
Blackwell Science, Inc.
Commerce Place
350 Main Street
Malden, MA 02148 5018
(*Orders:*   Tel: 800 759 6102
                          781 388 8250
                Fax: 781 388 8255)

Canada
Login Brothers Book Company
324 Saulteaux Crescent
Winnipeg, Manitoba R3J 3T2
(*Orders:*   Tel: 204 837-2987
                Fax: 204 837-3116)

Australia
Blackwell Science Pty Ltd
54 University Street
Carlton, Victoria 3053
(*Orders:*   Tel: 03 9347 0300
                Fax: 03 9347 5001)

A catalogue record for this title is available from the British Library

ISBN 0-632-05216-3

Library of Congress Cataloging-in-Publication Data
Martin, Mike W. S.
    Small animal ECGs: an introductory guide/Mike Martin.
        p.   cm.
    Includes bibliographical references (p.   ).
    ISBN 0-632-05216-3
    1. Veterinary electrocardiography. I. Title.
SF811.M37   1999
636.089′61207547—dc21   99-40470
                                          CIP

For further information on Blackwell Science, visit our website:
www.blackwell-science.com

Dedication

To my family: my wife Mary

and our three sons, David, Dennis and Sean

Contents

Contents

Preface

The aim of this guide is to provide an introduction to electrocardiography for anyone embarking on this subject. It has been written in such a way (I hope) that it is easy to understand. In part, it has been adapted and developed from frequent lecturing on this topic and feedback by audience interaction. This has resulted in a method of teaching electrocardiography that appears to have succeeded in providing the basis for understanding. Whether this transfers to a book remains to be seen, but I have deliberately used a number of diagrams to illustrate the points being made. Once this book has been read, the reader hopefully will be enthused and enlightened enough to proceed to more advanced ECG textbooks – a further reading list is given at the end. This book should not be used as a reference guide, but simply a stepping stone to such texts.

The book has been written in the expectation that the reader will read it from beginning to end, rather than try to pick out a chapter to read. I think that anyone who is new to ECGs will finding reading it from the beginning the easiest way to grasp the concepts of electrocardiography. In trying to keep this book as an introductory guide, I have (deliberately) not provided a comprehensive list of arrhythmias. In doing so I have had to decide which rhythm disturbances to leave out and which to keep in. This has been a difficult task! On balance I suspect even more rhythm disturbances and abnormalities should have been left out, such as intraventricular conduction disturbances. However, as these are occasionally seen in practice, I have therefore included them, although at the very end of the book!

Having said all that, I hope you, the reader, will find this an enjoyable and easy read, whilst also educational.

Mike Martin

Acknowledgements

I would like to thank all those who have assisted in production of this book, from those in the audience during lectures who provided feedback, to colleagues who have helped in reading (scrutineering and editing) the book during its embryogenesis, particularly Mary Martin and Anne Marie Taffs.

About the author

Mike Martin qualified from Dublin Veterinary School in 1986. He worked for two years in mixed practice and four years at the Royal (Dick) School of Veterinary Studies, University of Edinburgh, as a Housephysician and a Resident in Veterinary Cardiology, during which time he gained the Certificate and then Diploma in Veterinary Cardiology. He then moved to private referral practice with the formation of Godiva Referrals in Coventry for four years. During that time he gained Specialist status in Cardiology. In 1997 he founded the Veterinary Cardiorespiratory Centre in Kenilworth, Warwickshire which is a referral-only practice. He also runs a transtelephonic ECG service in the UK and Ireland, and provides an ECG and radiography interpretation service for practitioners.

Mike is an active and well recognised clinician, he has produced a number of publications and is a frequently invited speaker at meetings and courses. He has been an examiner for the RCVS Certificate and Diploma, and he has been past Honorary Secretary of the Veterinary Cardiovascular Society. He is co-author of the book *Cardiorespiratory diseases of the dog and cat* which is also published by Blackwell Science and is a recipient of the BSAVA Dunkin Award.

PART 1
Understanding the electricity of the heart and how it produces an ECG complex

1 • What is an ECG?

An **electrocardiograph** (**ECG**), in its simplest form, is a voltmeter (or galvanometer) that records the changing electrical activity in the heart by means of positive and negative electrodes (Fig. 1.1). **Electrocardiography** is the process of recording these changing potential differences.

While a positive (+ve) and negative (−ve) electrode can be placed almost anywhere on, or in, the body to record electrical changes, one of the most common and simplest methods is to place these electrodes on the limbs of the animal – referred to as a **body surface limb ECG recording**. In comparison, for example, electrodes can be placed on the chest (precordial chest ECG recording – very commonly used in humans) or inside the cardiac chambers (for electrophysiological studies). This book is confined to the limb ECG recording, the most commonly used method in veterinary medicine.

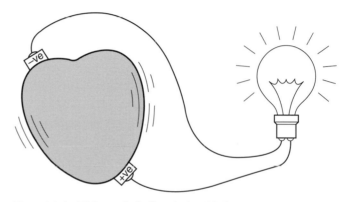

Figure 1.1 An ECG records the 'heart's electricity'.

3

2 • The electricity of the heart

For the heart to function efficiently as a 'pump system' it must have a co-ordinated contraction, the two atria contracting and passing blood into the two ventricles, followed by contraction of the ventricles that push blood out of the heart and into the aorta and pulmonary artery, i.e. there must be a co-ordinated atrioventricular contraction. In order for the cardiac muscle cells to contract, they must first receive an electrical stimulus. It is this electrical activity that is detected by an ECG.

The electrical stimulus must first depolarise the two atria. Then, with an appropriate time interval, stimulate the two ventricles. The heart must then repolarise (and 'refill') in time for the next stimulus and contraction. Additionally, it must repeatedly do so, increasing in rate with an increase in demand and conversely, slowing at rest.

Formation of the normal P–QRS–T complex

While all cells within the heart have the potential to generate their own electrical activity, the **sinoatrial (SA) node** is the fastest part of the electrical circuit to do so and is therefore the 'rate controller', termed the **pacemaker**. The rate of the SA node is influenced by the balance in autonomic tone, i.e. the

sympathetic (increases rate) and parasympathetic (decreases rate) systems.

The electrical discharge for each cardiac cycle (Fig. 2.1) starts

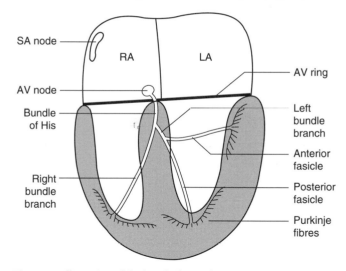

Figure 2.1 Illustration of the heart's electrical circuit. SA – sinoatrial; AV – atrioventricular; RA – right atrium; LA – left atrium.

in the SA node. Depolarisation spreads through the atrial muscle cells. The depolarisation wave then spreads through the **atrioventricular (AV) node**, but it does so relatively slower, creating a delay. Conduction passes through the AV ring (from the atria into the ventricles) through a narrow pathway called the **bundle of His**. This then divides in the ventricular septum into **left and right bundle branches** (going to the left and right ventricles). The left bundle branch divides further into **anterior and posterior fascicles**. The conduction tissue spreads into the myocardium as very fine branches called **Purkinje fibres**.

Formation of the P wave

The SA node is therefore the start of the electrical depolarisation wave. This depolarisation wave spreads through the atria (somewhat like the ripples in water created by dropping a stone). As the parts of the atria nearest the SA node are depolarised, this creates an electrical **potential difference** between depolarised atria and parts not yet depolarised (i.e. still in a resting state).

If a negative (−ve) and positive (+ve) electrode were placed approximately in line with that shown on the diagram (Fig. 2.2), then this would result in the voltmeter (i.e. the ECG machine) detecting the depolarisation wave travelling from the SA node, across the atria, in the general direction of the +ve electrode. On the ECG recording, all positive deflections are displayed as an upward (i.e. positive) deflection on the ECG paper, and negative deflections are displayed downwards. The

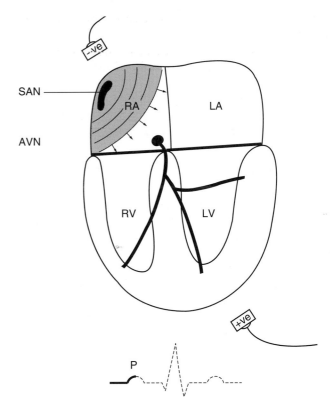

Figure 2.2 Illustration of partial depolarisation of the atria and formation of the P wave. The shaded area represents depolarised myocardial cells and the arrows, the direction in which the depolarisation wave in travelling. RA – right atrium; LA – left atrium; RV – right ventricle; LV – left ventricle; SAN – sinoatrial node; AVN – atrioventricular node.

atrial depolarisation wave therefore creates an upward excursion of the stylus on the ECG paper.

When the whole of the atria become depolarised then there is no longer an electrical potential difference and thus the stylus returns to its idle position – referred to as the **baseline**. The brief upward deflection of the stylus on the ECG paper creates the P wave, representing atrial electrical activity (Fig. 2.3). The muscle mass of the atria is fairly small and thus the electrical changes associated with depolarisation are also small.

The P–R interval

During the course of atrial depolarisation, the AV node also becomes depolarised. However, the speed with which the electrical depolarisation wave travels through the AV node is deliberately slow so that ventricular contraction will be correctly co-ordinated following atrial contraction. Once the depolarisation wave passes through the AV node, it travels very rapidly through the specialised conduction tissues of the ventricles, i.e. the bundle of His, the left and right bundle branches and Purkinje fibres.

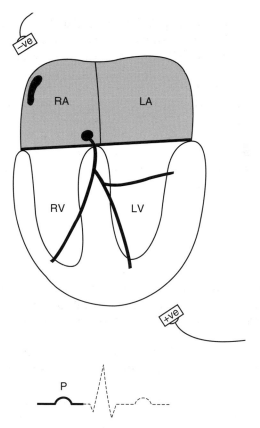

Figure 2.3 Illustration of complete depolarisation of the atria and formation of the P wave. RA – right atrium; LA – left atrium; RV – right ventricle; LV – left ventricle.

The formation of the QRS complex

The Q waves

Initially the first part of the ventricles to depolarise is the ventricular septum, with a small depolarisation wave which travels in a direction away from the +ve electrode (Fig. 2.4). This creates a small downward, or negative, deflection on the ECG paper – termed the Q wave.

The R wave

Then the bulk of the ventricular myocardium is depolarised. This creates a depolarisation wave that travels towards the +ve electrode (Fig. 2.5). As it is a large mass of muscle tissue it usually creates a large deflection – this is termed the R wave.

The S wave

Following depolarisation of the majority of the ventricles, the only remaining parts are basilar portions. This creates a depolarisation wave that travels away from the +ve electrode and is a small mass of tissue (Fig. 2.6). Thus, this creates a small negative deflection on the ECG paper – the S wave.

While the different parts of the QRS waveform can be identified, it is often easier to think of the whole ventricular depolarisation waveform as the QRS complex. This will avoid confusion of the correct and proper naming of the different parts of the QRS complex.

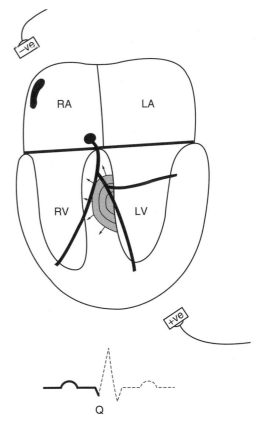

Figure 2.4 Illustration of depolarisation of the ventricular septum and formation of the Q wave. RA – right atrium; LA – left atrium; RV – right ventricle; LV – left ventricle.

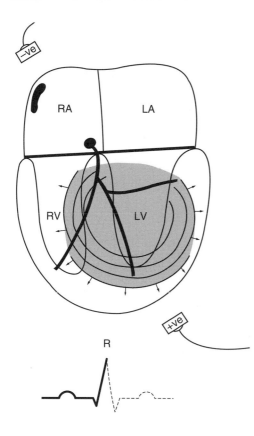

Figure 2.5 Illustration of depolarisation of the bulk of the ventricular myocardium and formation of the R wave. RA – right atrium; LA – left atrium; RV – right ventricle; LV – left ventricle.

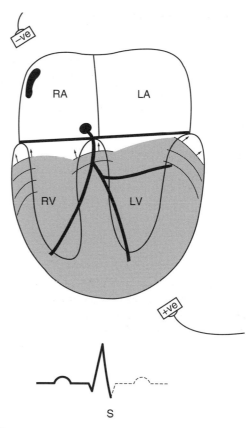

Figure 2.6 Illustration of depolarisation of the basilar portions of the ventricles and formation of the S wave. RA – right atrium; LA – left atrium; RV – right ventricle; LV – left ventricle.

Nomenclature of the QRS complex

The different parts of the QRS complex are labelled strictly as follows:

- The first downward deflection is called the Q wave; it always precedes the R wave.
- Any upward deflection is called the R wave; it may or may not be preceded by a Q wave.
- Any downward deflection after an R wave is called an S wave; regardless of whether there is a Q wave or not.

Having explained this, it is much easier to think of the 'QRS complex' as a whole, rather than to try to recognise its individual parts.

The T wave

Following complete depolarisation (and contraction) of the ventricles they then repolarise in time for the next stimulus. This phase of repolarisation creates a potential difference across the ventricular myocardium, until it is completely repolarised. This results in a deflection from the baseline – termed the T wave (Fig. 2.7).

The T wave in dogs and cats is very variable, it can be negative or positive or even biphasic (i.e. a bit of both). This is because repolarisation of the myocardium in small animals is a little random, unlike humans, for example, in which repolarisation is very organised and always results in a positive T wave. Thus, the diagnostic value obtainable from abnor-

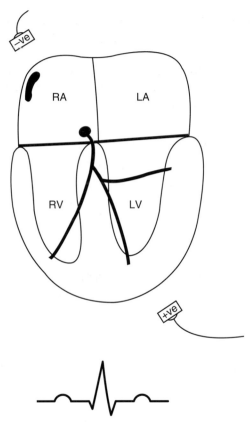

Figure 2.7 Illustration of complete depolarisation and repolarisation of the ventricles and completion of the P–QRS–T complex. RA – right atrium; LA – left atrium; RV – right ventricle; LV – left ventricle.

malities in the T wave of small animals is very limited, unlike the very useful features of abnormal T waveforms seen in humans.

The repolarisation wave of the atria (T_a) is rarely recognised on a surface ECG, as it is very small and is usually hidden within the QRS complex.

Rhythms of sinus origin

The formation of the normal ECG complex has been explained above; this normal complex is termed a **sinus complex**. A sequence of beats originating from the SA node will form a sinus rhythm, four common sinus rhythms are described below.

Sinus rhythm

The stimulus originates regularly at a constant rate from the SA node (dominant pacemaker) depolarising the atria and ventricles normally producing a co-ordinated atrioventricular contraction.

ECG characteristics

There is a normal P wave followed by normal QRS–T waves. The rhythm is regular (constant) and the rate is within normal for age and breed (Fig. 2.8).

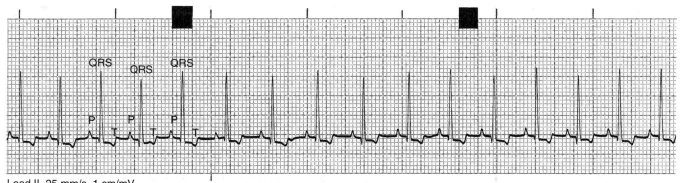

Lead II, 25 mm/s, 1 cm/mV

Figure 2.8 ECG from a dog showing a normal sinus rhythm at a rate of 140/min.

The size of the ECG complexes are typically small in cats (Fig. 2.9). Obtaining an artifact-free tracing is therefore important (in cats) to identify clearly the ECG complexes.

Clinical significance
This is a normal rhythm.

Sinus arrhythmia

The stimulus originates from the SA node, but the rate varies (increases and decreases) regularly. This is associated with the variation in autonomic tone which is often synchronous with respiration and sometimes therefore called **respiratory sinus arrhythmia.**

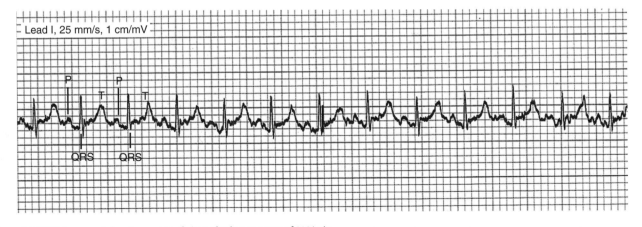

Figure 2.9 ECG from a cat showing a normal sinus rhythm at a rate of 220/min.

ECG characteristics

There is a normal P wave followed by normal QRS–T waves. The rhythm varies in rate; often associated with respiration (Fig. 2.10). The rhythm can sometimes be described as being regularly irregular, i.e. the variation in rate is fairly regular. The rate is within normal for age and breed.

Clinical significance

This is a normal and common rhythm in dogs. It is associated with an increase in parasympathetic activity (i.e. vagal tone) on the SA node. There is commonly a regular variation in rate often associated with respiration (i.e. it speeds up and slows down). Since sinus arrhythmia is an indicator of increased parasympathetic tone, conversely, it is also an indicator of reduced sympathetic tone. In dogs with heart failure one of the compensatory responses is an increase in sympathetic tone and therefore normal sinus arrhythmia is often lost and a sinus tachycardia develops. Sinus arrhythmia is uncommon in the cat and it might be seen in association with dyspnoea.

Sinus tachycardia

The SA node generates an impulse and depolarisation that are faster than normal.

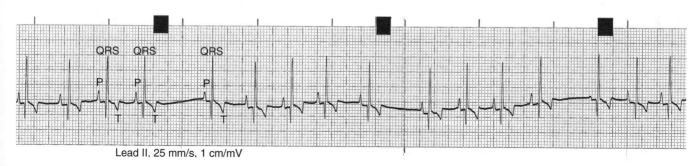

Lead II, 25 mm/s, 1 cm/mV

Figure 2.10 ECG from a dog showing a normal respiratory sinus arrhythmia at a rate of 110/min.

ECG characteristics

There is a normal sinus rhythm but at a faster rate than normal (Fig. 2.11).

Clinical significance

Sinus tachycardia is a non-specific rhythm disturbance. Although it is often seen in heart failure, caused by a compensatory sympathetic drive, it is often due to a physiological response such as stress, excitement and fear. Thus, it is of paramount importance to evaluate the 'state' of the patient – which during an ECG recording may, of course, cause a degree of stress and fear! Comparing the heart rate obtained during physical examination, when the animal is relaxed, is therefore invaluable in assessing its significance. Sinus tachycardia can also be as a result of a disease process such as pyrexia, pain, anaemia, shock, dehydration, haemorrhage, septicaemia, toxaemia, hyperthyroidism. Current medication, sedatives or anaesthetics should also be taken into consideration.

Sinus bradycardia

The SA node generates an impulse and depolarisation slower

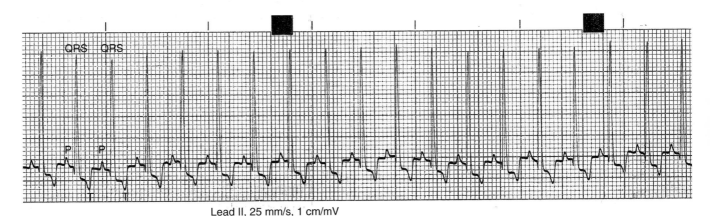

Lead II, 25 mm/s, 1 cm/mV

14

Figure 2.11 ECG from 13-year-old Cavalier King Charles spaniel dog in heart failure due to mitral valve disease. There is a sinus tachycardia at 180/min.

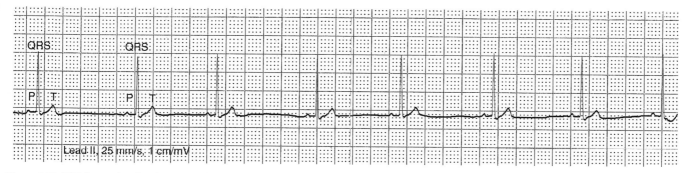

Figure 2.12 ECG from a dog showing a sinus bradycardia at 65/min.

than normal. This can be a normal feature in some giant-breed dogs and in athletically fit animals.

ECG characteristics

There is a normal sinus rhythm but at a slower rate than normal (Fig. 2.12).

Clinical significance

Sinus bradycardia could be due to hypothyroidism, hyper-kalaemia, hypothermia, elevated intracranial pressure (e.g. following cranial trauma), systemic disease (e.g. renal failure) or drugs (tranquillisers or anti-arrhythmic drugs). Cats, paradoxically, sometimes present with a sinus bradycardia when in heart failure (since one of the compensatory responses to heart failure is an increase in sympathetic tone, a tachycardia would be expected).

3 • Abnormal electricity of the heart

Dysrhythmia literally means abnormal rhythm; arrhythmia is a synonymous term. Dysrhythmias include abnormalities in rate, abnormalities associated with ectopia and those associated with abnormalities in conduction. Dysrhythmias that are essentially slow are referred to as **bradydysrhythmias**, and those that are fast as **tachydysrhythmias**.

First identify the morphology of the normal QRS complex

Chapter 2 explained the formation of a normal sinus complex. It is important when examining an ECG tracing to identify (from the ECG recording) a normal sinus complex for that animal. Note the shape of the ventricular depolarisation and repolarisation waves, i.e. the QRS complex and T wave. To produce this shape of QRS–T, then depolarisation of the ventricles has occurred by conduction from (or through) the AV node, i.e. ventricular depolarisation has been initiated from the AV node (see Chapter 2). It is of paramount importance in any tracing, especially if there are a variety of shapes of QRS complexes, to determine which shape represents conduction that has arisen (correctly) via the AV node.

The morphology of an ectopic ventricular depolarisation

Any QRS–T complex, therefore, that is of a different shape (from the QRS–T of a normal sinus complex) represents an abnormal beat. When the QRS–T complex is different from the normal sinus complex, the only possible site of origin is a ventricular ectopic focus – there is nowhere else that can stimulate the ventricles except a ventricular ectopic. Additionally these ventricular ectopic complexes are not associated with a preceding P wave.

From Fig. 3.1 it can be seen that the direction of ventricular depolarisation is different to the direction that would have occurred from depolarisation arising from the AV node (cf. Figs 2.4–2.6). In this example the ventricular ectopic depolarisation wave is away from the +ve electrode and therefore displayed on the ECG paper as below the baseline, i.e. the QRS complex is negative. Secondly, because conduction has not travelled through the normal (therefore fast) electrical conduction tissue (it has depolarised the ventricular muscle mass from 'cell to cell') the time it takes to depolarise the ventricles is prolonged. Thus, not only is the QRS complex of the ventricular ectopic different in shape, but it is also prolonged (it takes a longer time). Quite often the T wave following the QRS complex of a ventricular ectopic is opposite and large in shape to the QRS.

Ventricular ectopic complexes can arise from any part of the ventricles and thus the direction in which they depolarise the ventricles is variable. To put it another way: since the direction in which the depolarisation wave travels in relation to the +ve electrode is variable, the shape and magnitude of the QRS complex of a ventricular complex will also be variable (Fig. 3.2).

The important point is that the QRS of a ventricular ectopic complex is different to the QRS complex of one that has arisen from the AV node and travelled normally down the electrical conducting tissue to the ventricles.

A ventricular ectopic complex can occur quickly (or early) and is therefore termed a **ventricular *premature* complex.** If

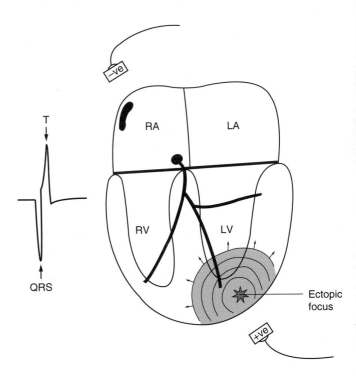

Figure 3.1 Diagram illustrating an ectopic focus with the spreading out of the depolarisation wave (*left*), and the formation of a QRS–T complex (*right*) associated with the ventricular ectopic. RA – right atrium; LA – left atrium; RV – right ventricle; LV – left ventricle.

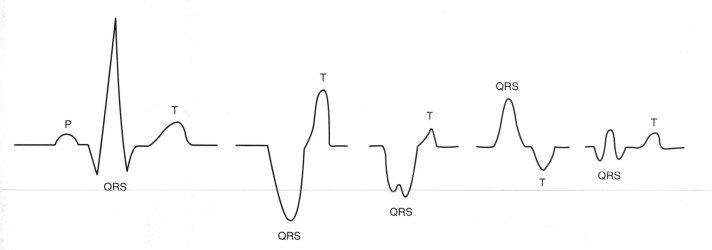

Figure 3.2 Illustration of a normal complex (first complex), followed by four examples of QRS–T complexes with an abnormal morphology due to ventricular ectopic depolarisations. It is paramount to identify the morphology of the QRS complex associated with a sinus complex (first complex). Any QRS complexes of a different morphology (for that animal) must arise from an ectopic ventricular focus.

a ventricular ectopic occurs after a pause (or with delay) then is it referred to as a **ventricular *escape* complex** (Fig. 3.3).

The morphology of an ectopic supraventricular depolarisation

Any ectopic stimuli arising above the ventricles are referred to as supraventricular (Fig. 3.4). These can be divided into two categories: (1) those occurring in atrial muscle mass (atrial ectopics) and (2) those arising from within the AV node (junctional or nodal ectopics).

No matter where supraventricular ectopics arise, they must travel down the normal His–Purkinje tissue and depolarise the ventricles as normal. Thus, the morphology of the QRS com-

plex associated with a supraventricular ectopic is normal, i.e. the same as the QRS complex for a sinus complex. This means that the identification of a supraventricular ectopic can be difficult. In the vast majority of cases however, it occurs as a premature beat, and so it is primarily recognised by its premature timing (Fig. 3.5).

While the timing (in relation to its QRS complex) and the morphology of the P wave (which is usually different from the normal P wave) can aid in identifying whether the ectopic arose from the atria (**atrial premature complex**) or the AV node (referred to as a **junctional or nodal premature complex**) it is of little practical importance in small animals until studying advanced ECGs. Additionally it does not affect the management or treatment in the vast majority of cases in small

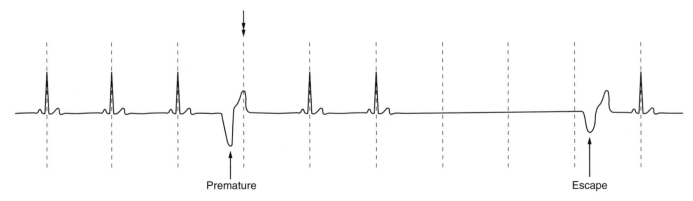

Premature

Escape

Figure 3.3 Illustration of (1) a ventricular premature complex (the double-headed arrow indicates the timing of when the next normal sinus complex would have occurred) and (2) a ventricular escape beat which occurred following a pause in the rhythm.

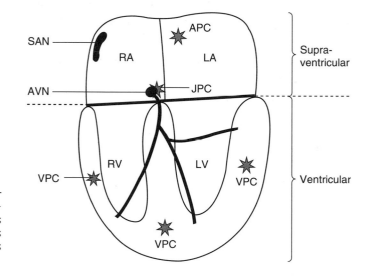

Figure 3.4 (*right*) Illustration of the origin of supraventricular and ventricular ectopic complexes. SAN – sinoatrial node; AVN – atrioventricular node; APC – atrial premature complex; JPC – junctional premature complex; VPC – ventricular premature complex; RA – right atrium; LA – left atrium; RV – right ventricle; LV – left ventricle.

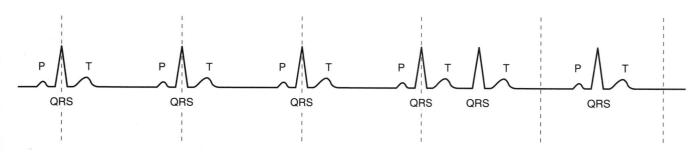

Figure 3.5 (*above*) Illustration of a supraventricular premature complex (fifth beat).

animals. Therefore, distinguishing between atrial and junctional premature complexes will not be discussed in this book, but referred to by the broader term of **supraventricular premature complexes.**

Mean electrical axis

Although depolarisation waves spread through the heart in 'all directions', the average direction and magnitude is represented by the QRS complex. If the QRS is predominantly positive (upwards), the average direction of the depolarisation waves is towards the +ve electrode. Conversely, if it is predominantly negative (downwards) then the depolarisation wave is moving away from the +ve electrode. When the QRS complex is equally positive and negative (and usually also small) then the depolarisation wave is moving at right angles to the +ve electrode.

The limb leads 'look at' the heart from six different directions. The average direction and magnitude of the depolarisation wave through the ventricles is termed the mean electrical axis (MEA) or the cardiac axis. As can be seen from Fig. 3.6, in which there is a normal axis, leads I, II, III and aVF have positive deflections and aVR and aVL are negative.

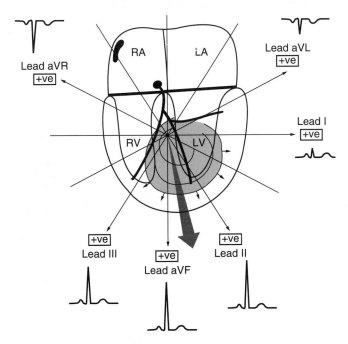

Figure 3.6 A normal mean electrical axis (large shaded arrow) and how this is 'seen' from the six limb leads. RA – right atrium; LA – left atrium; RV – right ventricle; LV – left ventricle.

Right axis deviation

If the right ventricle becomes enlarged as illustrated (either with hypertrophy or dilation), then the MEA swings to the right, because the large increase in muscle mass on the right side creates a large electrical potential difference during depolarisation.

In Fig. 3.7, for example, leads III and aVR become large and positive. Leads I, II and aVL become negative. Lead aVF is isoelectric in this example. This is termed a right axis deviation.

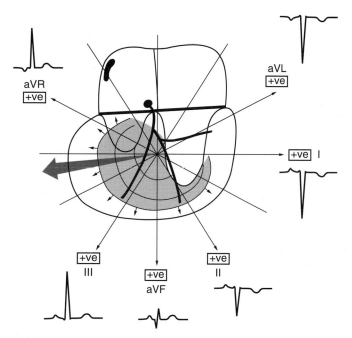

Figure 3.7 The mean electrical axis (large shaded arrow) in an animal with right ventricular enlargement (RVE) and how this is 'seen' from the six limb leads.

Left axis deviation

If the left ventricle becomes enlarged (either by hypertrophy or dilation), then the MEA swings to the left, because the large increase in muscle mass on the left side creates a large electrical potential difference during depolarisation.

In Fig. 3.8, for example, lead I becomes taller than lead II. Lead aVL is also positive. Leads III and aVR are negative and aVF is isoelectric. This is termed a left axis deviation.

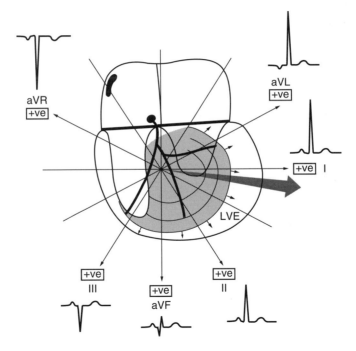

Figure 3.8 The mean electrical axis (large shaded arrow) in an animal with left ventricular enlargement (LVE) and how this is 'seen' from the six limb leads.

Eyeballing the mean electrical axis

With the foregoing illustrations, it can be seen that by examining whether lead I or lead III has the largest positive deflection, then the axis has swung towards lead I or III, thus there has been a left or right axis deviation, respectively.

By examining all six of the limb leads and finding the lead(s) with the largest positive deflection, the mean electrical axis must be approximately in the direction of that lead. Conversely, the largest negative deflection can also be used, in which case the mean electrical axis is in an approximate direction away from that lead. A quick, eyeballed, estimate of the mean electrical axis can therefore be made.

PART 2
The ECG machine explained, and how to use it!

4 • Bipolar lead systems

In Chapter 3, the +ve and −ve electrodes, in the diagrams, were placed so as to obtain a recording of the electricity of the heart. This *combination* of a +ve and −ve electrode is termed a **bipolar lead**, simply meaning between two poles, i.e. a +ve and a −ve pole (electrode). However, the term 'lead' can cause immense confusion, as an ECG cable or wire is often also called an ECG lead in common parlance. This potential confusion should be avoided. In 'ECG-speak', a lead is formed by a combination of a −ve and +ve electrode placed on the body.

While there are usually four ECG cables or wires (I'll avoid 'lead' here!), one of these is an earth. The other three are the active cables to which the −ve and +ve electrodes are connected. All cables are labelled and/or colour coded for identification, to ensure correct placement on each of the limbs.

When the ECG cables are then attached to the animal, switching 'channels' on the ECG machine can provide different bipolar leads as shown in Fig. 4.1 on page 31. Thus, it can be seen how three ECG cables and electrodes can provide a total combination of six bipolar leads.

Table 4.1 ECG cable colour coding

Limb	Standard	American	Labelling often on medical ECG machines
Right fore	Red	White	RA (right arm)
Left fore	Yellow	Black	LA (left arm)
Left hind	Green	Red	LL (left leg)
Right hind (earth)	Black	Green	RL (right leg)

Occasionally, I receive ECGs from students with only the first four leads recorded (i.e. I, II, III and aVR). On enquiring as to why the other two leads (aVL and aVF) were not recorded I am told: 'because there are only four leads on the ECG machine'. That confusing term again! There are four cables, one is an earth and the other three are active, these three provide a combination of six bipolar leads.

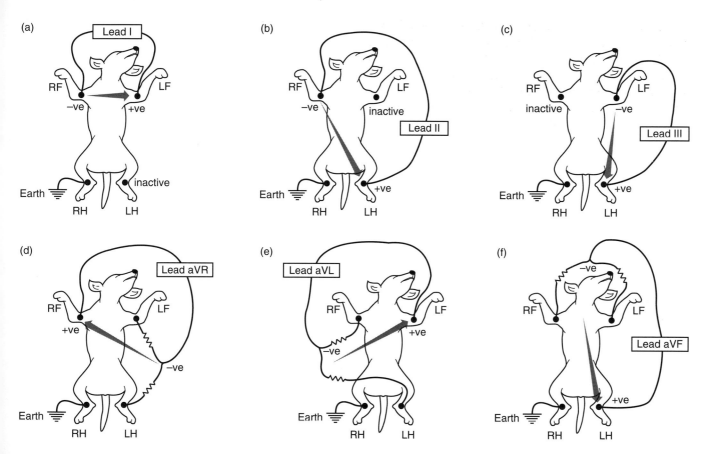

Figure 4.1 These diagrams illustrate how the six limb leads are generated by switching the electrode connections.

5 • Recording an ECG

The connectors (electrodes)

To connect the ECG cable to the animal's skin requires a connector – this is called an **electrode**. Since animals have a coat of hair, the commonly used human sticky adhesive electrodes (Fig. 5.1) are not convenient for everyday regular use. This is because a patch of hair would have to be shaved, the adhesive electrode applied and it still usually does not stick to animal skin! Therefore, it needs to be held in place by wrapping a bandage around the limb and electrode.

There are small metal plate electrodes – paediatric limb electrodes (Fig. 5.2), that can be used instead of crocodile clips, but need to be positioned on the limb by means of tape (Fig. 5.12), bandage or rubber band.

The most commonly used electrode to connect the ECG cable to the animal's skin is a crocodile clip (Fig. 5.3). While these provide an excellent electrical connection, their bite can be painful to less stoical animals. To minimise the pain of crocodile clips the teeth can be filed down a little and the clips bent outwards (until they are atraumatic but still stay in place). Or a small conductive plate can be soldered into the tip of the teeth.

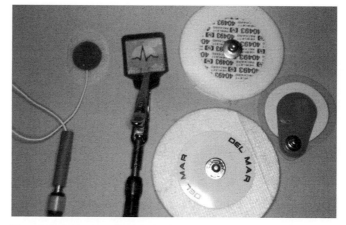

Figure 5.1 A selection of 'human' adhesive electrodes.

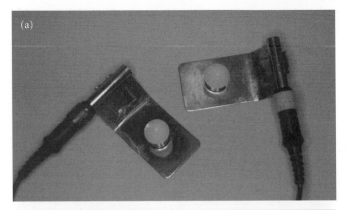

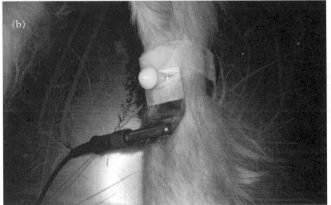

Figure 5.2 (a) 'Human' paediatric limb electrodes; and (b) how an electrode can be attached with tape to the leg of an animal (the hair usually needs to be clipped to ensure good contact and gel used between the electrode and skin).

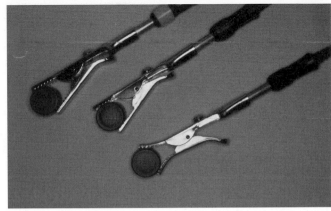

Figure 5.3 Crocodile clips commonly used in animals. The middle one has had its teeth filed down and the lower one also bent outwards – these are method to soften the bite on this type of electrode.

Making the connection

This is the single most important part of ECG recording to obtain a good diagnostic quality tracing. Since crocodile clips are the most commonly used form of electrodes, the following discussion will be based on these. But if you have decided to use an alternative electrode, then adapt the description accordingly.

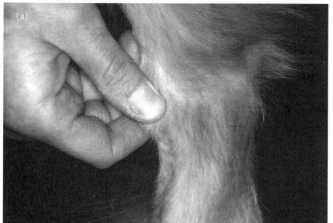

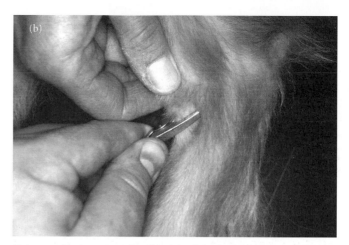

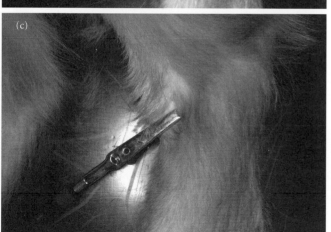

Figure 5.4 Placing a crocodile clip to the skin of a dog (flexor angle of hock in this instance). Pinch a good piece of skin (a), position the crocodile clip with its jaws fully open and over the skin as far as possible (b), so that the clips maintains a good bite of skin (c) and therefore good clip–skin contact.

Using spirit

It is often sufficient with crocodile clips to pick up a fold of skin between finger and thumb (rolling the skin to feel its edge through a hairy coat) and with the other hand open the crocodile clip maximally, part the hair and attach the clip to the skin (Fig. 5.4). To obtain good conduction between skin and crocodile clip requires the addition of a conducting medium – spirit is often adequate. Spray with a little spirit (or alcohol),

35

just sufficient to wet the crocodile clip and through the hair to the skin.

However, spirit evaporates after 5–10 min, so this method would not suffice if the ECG recording takes longer than this (such as during anaesthetic monitoring). Additionally, if spirit does not produce a good-quality, artifact-free recording, then an alternative method needs to be considered.

Using gel

Shave the site where the crocodile clip is to be placed. Either: (1) rub a little gel (ECG gel is ideal, but ultrasound gel or K-Y jelly are cheap alternatives) on to the skin (Fig. 5.5) and then attach the crocodile clip as above; or (2) attach the crocodile clips then rub the gel on the clip and around it onto the skin (Fig. 5.6). This 'way round' is usually easier, as your fingers are not too slippery to open the crocodile clips thereafter!

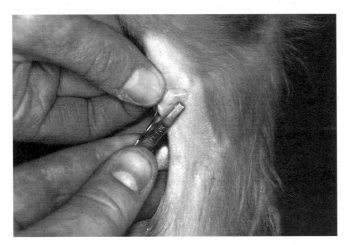

Figure 5.5 Gel can be applied to the skin before placement of the crocodile clip.

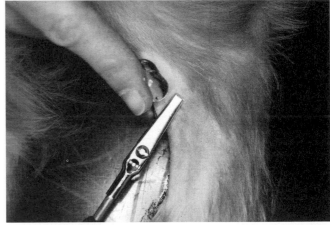

Figure 5.6 Alternatively gel can be applied after the crocodile has been attached, over the clip and adjacent skin.

Where to place the electrodes

The site of attachment of the electrodes is on each of the four limbs, using the correct ECG cable on the correct leg – as labelled (see the colour coding given in Table 4.1). Where exactly on the leg is not too critical. Essentially a good loose fold of skin is required preferably with little hair. In each animal you need to pinch the skin at various sites on the limbs to find the best site.

Forelegs

In the author's experience, the flexor angle of the elbow is a useful site (Fig. 5.7).

An alternative site is caudal and just dorsal to the elbow. However, since this is close to the chest, respiratory movement can result in movement of the cable and clip, thus the ECG recording may be spoiled by movement artifact. Another site is halfway between the elbow and carpus, on the palmer aspect of the leg.

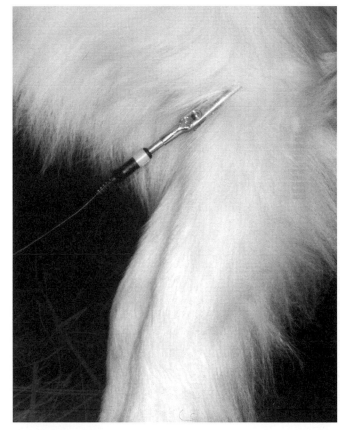

Figure 5.7 A useful site of attachment for the crocodile clips on the forelimbs is the skin at the flexor angle of the elbow.

Hind legs

In the author's experience, the flexor angle of the hock (or sometimes just above this) is a useful site (Fig. 5.8). Alternative sites are either above or below the knee, on the dorsal aspect of the limb.

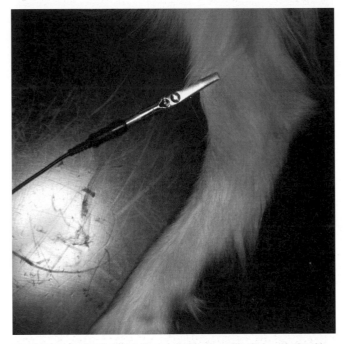

Figure 5.8 A useful site of attachment for the crocodile clips on the hind legs is the skin at the flexor angle of the hock.

When using adhesive electrodes

Adhesive electrodes usually need to be held in place by a bandage, therefore shave sites on the forelegs above the carpus and on the hind legs above or below the hock (Fig. 5.9).

Adhesive electrodes can also be placed on the central pad (of the paw) in small animals (Fig. 5.10) – this provides a satisfactory site of contact, although instability of the electrode can result in some movement artifact. This can be a useful site in other domestic small and exotic animals seen by the veterinary practitioner.

Isolating the electrodes

Once all the electrodes have been attached it is essential to ensure that each electrode, the skin to which it is attached and the conducting medium (e.g. the spirit or gel), are not touching any other part of the animal, the handler or the table. This has the potential to cause electrical shorting and introduce artifacts into the ECG recording.

How to position the ECG cables

In addition to the above, it is prudent not to place the crocodile clips such that the ECG cable runs over the animal which can lead to respiratory movement artifact (as mentioned above) or to then twist the cable and ultimately the clip and

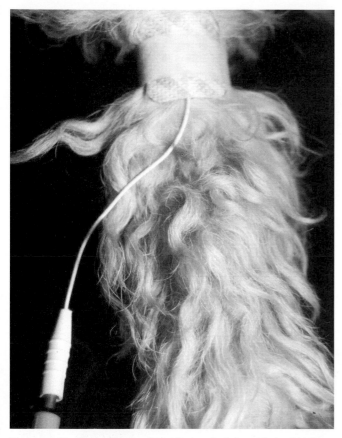

Figure 5.9 Placing an adhesive electrode on a dog's leg with the aid of tape to hold it in place.

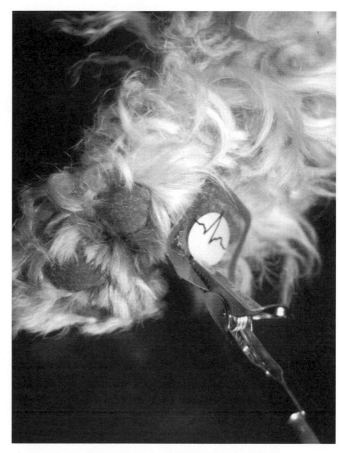

Figure 5.10 An adhesive electrode on the central pad of a foot.

skin – even stoical animals may not tolerate this. When applying the crocodile clip have the ECG cable positioned away from the animal (Fig. 5.11) and resting on the table (or ground).

Positioning the animal

To minimise the electrical activity of skeletal muscles the animal must be relaxed and resting. If the animal trembles, shakes,

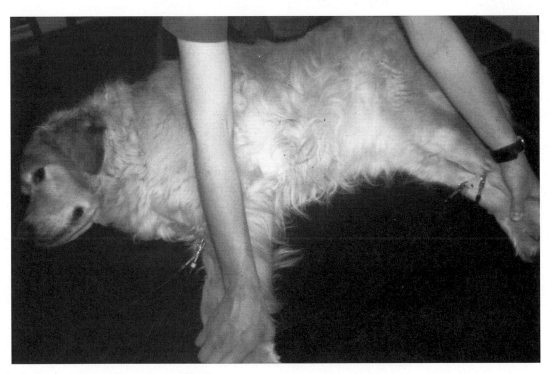

40   Figure 5.11 A dog having an ECG recording using crocodile clips.

pants or purrs, then all this activity will be manifest on the ECG resulting in baseline artifact. This may hide small ECG complexes such as P waves, especially in cats, or mimic ECG activity. Thus a good-quality ECG will have minimal movement and there should be a nice steady baseline in between each ECG complex.

If the animal would be put at risk (e.g. if it was in respiratory distress) by making it adopt a position (as follows) that it would not tolerate, then an ECG should be recorded in whatever position is achievable.

Dogs

Dogs are preferably placed in right lateral recumbency (Fig. 5.12). In many dogs a recumbent position will reduce skeletal muscle electrical activity. And the normal values for

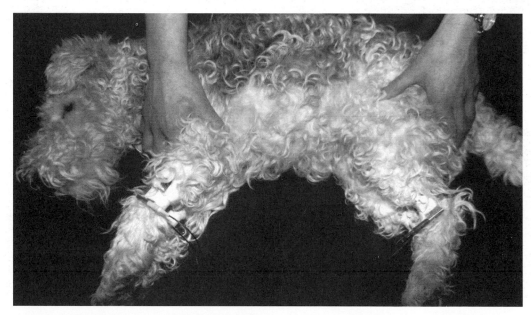

Figure 5.12 A dog having an ECG recording using paediatric limb electrodes.

the dog ECG have been determined based on this position. If measurement of amplitudes are not critical, such as when examining primarily an arrhythmia, then recording an ECG while the dog lies, sits or even stands is acceptable, provided a good-quality tracing with minimal baseline movement artifact can be obtained.

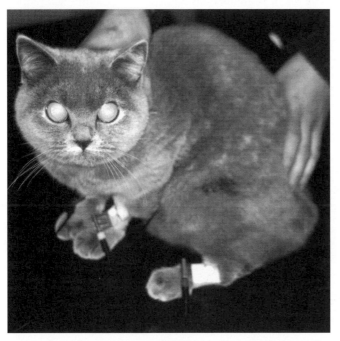

Figure 5.13 A cat having an ECG recording using paediatric limb electrodes.

42

Cats

The normal values for cats have not been determined in a lateral recumbent position, thus recumbent positioning is less important. Many cats will often sit in a hunched position quite still (Fig. 5.13) – but each individual cat is different and the veterinary surgeon must determine how each cat prefers to keep still. In fractious cats (if the electrodes can be placed!) putting the cat back in a basket together with the electrodes attached and ECG cables until it settles is a useful method. When, or if, the cat settles, the ECG can be recorded while the cats sits in the basket. However, this method should, of course, be aborted if the cats starts to bite the ECG cables. Often cats do resent the crocodile clips, in which case, shaving a patch of hair and bandaging in place adhesive electrodes or metal plates, although more time consuming, is easier!

Chemical restraint

All sedative and tranquilliser drugs have a variable effect on the heart and/or autonomic tone. Drugs can therefore change the rate and rhythm of the heart directly or through effects on the autonomic tone. So, if you are performing an ECG to determine what the arrhythmia is that you heard, then there is a possibility that this will change if a chemical restraint is used. Ideally, therefore, any form of chemical restraint should be avoided prior to recording an ECG. If chemical restraint cannot be avoided, then based on physical examination, determine the rate and rhythm before and after using the drugs, and any differences should be taken into account when interpreting the ECG recording.

Setting up and preparing the ECG machine

This will vary a little between different ECG machines and adjustments to the following guidelines (which are based on a standard ECG machine) should be allowed.

Paper speed

Select the paper speed. Options are usually 25 or 50 mm/s (Fig. 5.14), and sometimes 100 mm/s. The paper speed selec-tion is partly dependent on the animal's heart rate. As a guide: for normal heart rates in dogs set the speed at 25 mm/s, but if there is a fast heart rate (and routinely for cats) set the paper speed at 50 mm/s. In ECG machines with a computer-type print-out which produces a steppiness in the lines (i.e. pixel effect), measurement of ECG complex durations is best achieved at 100 mm/s.

Calibration

This is usually set at 1 cm/mV. However, if the complexes are very small this can be increased to 2 cm/mV and if the com-plexes are very large it can be reduced to 0.5 cm/mV. The

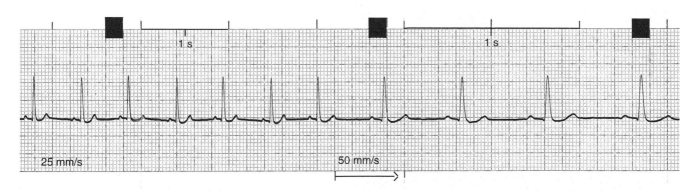

Figure 5.14 ECG showing the effect of paper speed.

calibration should be marked on the ECG paper by briefly running the ECG paper and pressing the 1 mV marker button (Fig. 5.15) – found on most standard ECG recorders.

Filter setting

Ideally, if good connections have been made, this can usually be left off, i.e. no filter. Additionally amplitude measurement should always be performed in an unfiltered tracing, as the dampening effect of the filter will reduce the amplitude of the complexes by a variable, although small, amount. If primari-

ly examining for an arrhythmia and there is baseline artifact that cannot seem to be avoided, then filtering can reduce the baseline artifact and make reading of the ECG tracing easier (Figs 5.16 and 6.2).

Positioning the stylus

During the recording the stylus should be positioned (if this is manually operated on the ECG machine) so that the whole of the ECG complex is within the 'graph lines' of the ECG paper. If the ECG produces particularly large complexes that

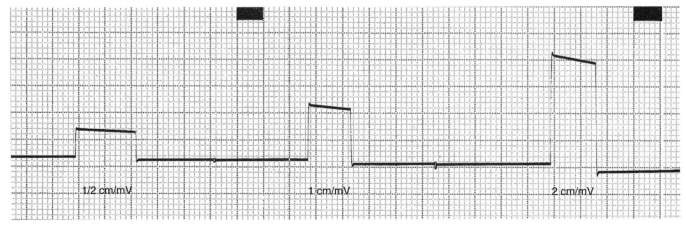

1/2 cm/mV   1 cm/mV   2 cm/mV

Figure 5.15 ECG showing three 1 mV calibrations marks at different sensitivity settings: 0.5, 1 and 2 cm/mV.

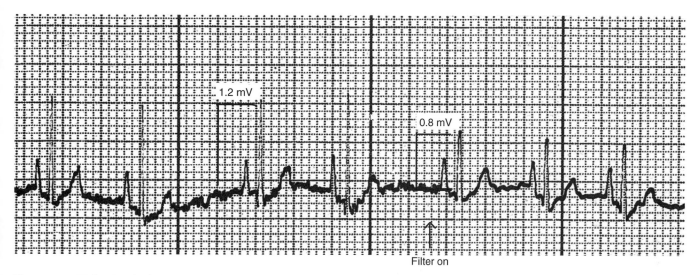

Figure 5.16 ECG showing the damping effect of the filter. Note the reduction in amplitude of the complexes (R waves from 1.2 to 0.8 mV) – measurements should be made from an unfiltered tracing to avoid potential underestimation of amplitudes. But also note the reduction in muscle tremor artifact (25 mm/s and 1 cm/mV).

run-off the 'graph paper' (or outside the limits of the stylus or paper) this is referred to as **clipping** (Fig. 5.17). Remember then to move the stylus, up or down, so that the whole of the ECG tracing is within the graph paper (and not extending into the white margins) or alternatively reduce the calibration – whichever is more appropriate.

Recording an ECG – a suggested routine

Ten seconds of all six limb leads

Run the ECG on each of the six bipolar leads, I, II, III, aVR, aVL and aVF, each for approximately 10 seconds. In order to ensure that each lead is well centred within the 'graph lines' of the ECG paper, briefly pause the ECG paper (with the stylus still moving) when switching the ECG machine from one lead to the next, until the stylus can be re-positioned as described above.

A rhythm strip

Switch back to lead II and record a long rhythm strip, 30–60 seconds, depending on each individual case requirement. If you have auscultated an occasional abnormal beat, then the ECG rhythm strip will need to be run until that abnormal beat is repeated. If lead II does not produce a good-

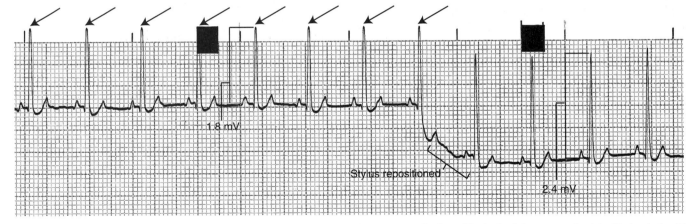

1.8 mV

Stylus repositioned

2.4 mV

Figure 5.17 ECG showing the effect of clipping (arrows). If this went unnoticed, the R wave amplitude could mistakenly be measured as 1.8 mV when it should have measured 2.4 mV – potentially a considerable underestimation.

quality tracing with satisfactorily large complexes, then run a rhythm strip on a lead that does. Or if you are searching for P waves (which can often be small and hard to see) then run the limb lead in which these are best shown.

A representative rhythm strip!

If you auscultated what you thought was an arrhythmia, but it is not revealed on the ECG rhythm strip, then simultaneously auscultate the animal while continuing to run the ECG recording. It might be that the abnormality is only intermittently present, in which case you may have to continue to auscultate the animal until the arrhythmia is heard and hopefully captured on ECG. Maybe the arrhythmia is still audible on auscultation but not recognised on the ECG – in this case the ECG tracing should be sent to a cardiologist for interpretation. Or, the abnormal heart sounds heard may not be an arrhythmia, but, for example, could be a gallop sound. In summary, ensure that the ECG recording obtained is representative of what you found on physical examination.

Label the tracing

Ensure the ECG recording is well labelled (unless the ECG machine does this automatically), either for future reference, or for other colleagues within your practice to be able to examine the recording, or in case you need to submit the tracing to a cardiologist for interpretation.

Checklist

- State in which position the animal was restrained.
- State if any chemical restraint was used.
- Note paper speed and if, and where, it was changed.
- Note calibration and if, and where, it was changed.
- Label filter level, and when, and where, it was used.
- Label each lead at its beginning.

6 • Artifacts

Artifacts are abnormal deflections reproduced on an ECG recording that are not associated with the electrical activity of the heart. They have the potential to either mask the ECG or mimic ECG activity: producing an artifact-free tracing is of paramount importance.

Electrical interference

Electrical interference produces fine, rapid and regular movements on the baseline of the ECG recording (Fig. 6.1). They are often associated with interference due to electrical cables (electromagnetic waves) within the room in which the recording is being made. They can be transmitted by the

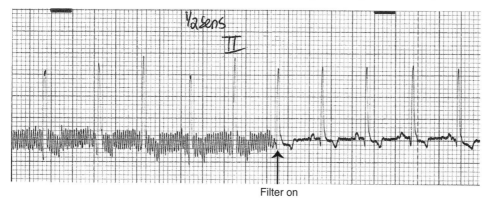

Filter on

Figure 6.1 ECG showing 50-cycle alternating current interference artifact (which masks the P waves on this example), which has then been removed by filtering (arrow) (25 mm/s and 0.5 cm/mV).

person restraining the animal who acts as an aerial or through the power-line of the ECG machine. The fine deflections usually occur at a rate of 50 per second (Hz) (60 per second in America).

To correct this problem:

- Ensure the clip-to-skin connections are good and are insulated (isolated), poor connections will permit electrical interference to manifest.
- Ensure the animal is insulated from the surface by placing a rug under it.
- Ensure the ECG machine is earthed (to the building), or try not to run on the mains supply but on battery.
- Try insulating the handler from the dog by having them wear gloves.

Muscle tremor artifact

This can look a little similar to electrical interference, but the fine deflections in this instance are not regular but fairly random. It can be produced by the animal trembling or shaking, or by trying to record the ECG in a standing animal (Fig. 6.2). Purring in a cat (Fig. 6.3) will also result in baseline 'trembling'!

To correct this problem:

- Ensure the limbs are relaxed and supported.
- Find a position in which the animal will relax best, preferably not standing.
- Try holding the limbs to minimise the tremor.
- To stop a cat purring: dab a little spirit on the cat's nose using cotton wool.

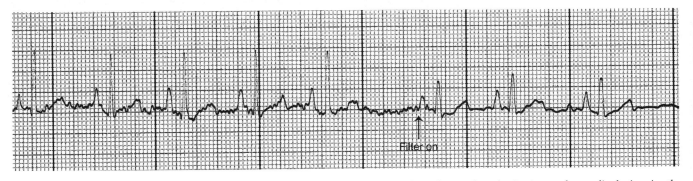

Figure 6.2 ECG showing muscle tremor artifact (see also Fig. 5.16), which is then filtered out (arrow). Note the reduction in complex amplitudes in using the filter (50 mm/s and 1 cm/mV).

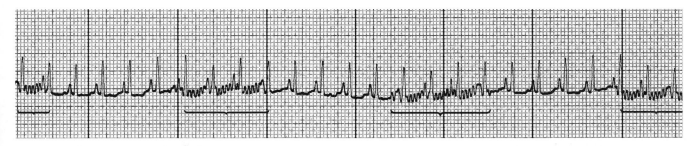

Figure 6.3 ECG from a cat with intermittent 'purring' artifact (brackets) (25 mm/s and 1 cm/mV).

Movement artifact

This is a more exaggerated form of tremor artifact, but in this case the deflections are not fine but variable and large. The stylus moves up and down the paper (Fig. 6.4a). It can be associated with respiratory movement (Fig. 6.4b) or if the animal is moving or struggling.

To correct this problem:

- Correction of this is similar to tremor artifact.
- Try to get the animal to relax and remain still.
- Ensure the ECG cables are not moving with movement of the animal, e.g. respiratory movement (see page 38), or because the clips are not stable and secure.

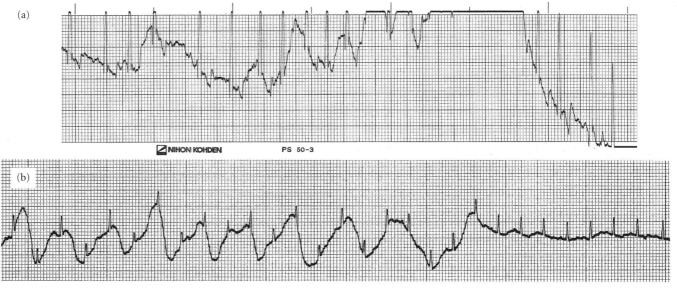

Figure 6.4 (a) ECG showing marked movement of the stylus due to movement or an unstable electrode (25 mm/s and 1 cm/mV). (b) ECG showing movement artifact synchronised with panting in a dog, which then stops panting towards the end of the recording (25 mm/s and 1 cm/mV).

Which leg moved?

With the aid of Figs 4.1(a–c) one can determine which leg is moving or causing connection problems. For example, if interference is seen in leads I and II, then the connection that is common to these leads is the right fore. Therefore, this connection needs to be checked and the connection improved or the leg held still. If interference is seen in leads I and III, then the left fore needs to be checked. And if interference is seen in leads II and III (Fig. 6.4c), then the left hind needs to be checked.

Incorrectly placed electrodes

This may result in inverted complexes or a bizarre mean electrical axis.

Tip: P waves are nearly always positive in leads I, II and III. Double check the position of the ECG cables, use the colour code chart in Table 4.1 if necessary.

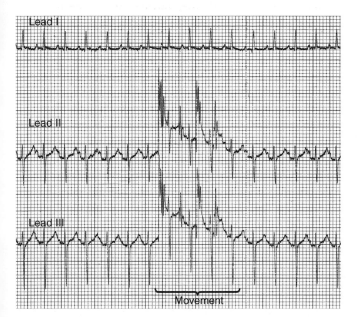

Figure 6.4 (c) ECG from a three-channel recording in a cat (with left anterior fascicular block – see later). Movement (bracketed) occurred in leads II and III which can be deduced to be movement of the left hind leg or its electrode – this is the connection that is common to these two leads (25 mm/s and 1 cm/mV).

7 • Approach to interpretation of the ECG recording

It is important to develop, and use, a routine when reading ECGs. Always read an ECG from its beginning, i.e. from left to right. When the ECG is difficult to read, start from the easiest part of the tracing that is recognisable, then continue reading (left to right) from that point.

It is important to not over-read or be too dependent on ECG findings. Since the ECG records only the electrical activity of the heart, it should be remembered that this limits the information that can be gained from it. It is often poorly related to the mechanical function of the heart and does not provide information about aetiology or severity of organic heart disease. A normal ECG does not necessarily infer the heart is normal, and likewise, an abnormal ECG is not necessarily indicative of heart disease. Additionally, if the ECG is abnormal, it is important to determine what the clinical significance is, and if treatment is indicated or not.

There are essentially four steps in ECG interpretation: rate, rhythm, complex measurement and mean electrical axis.

1. To calculate the heart rate (given as beats per minute)

This should be fairly easy, as you have already examined the animal and determined the heart rate on auscultation. (…?!)

The simplest method to calculate the rate from an ECG is to mark a 6-second strip of a representative part of the tracing. Count the number of complexes and multiply by 10. If the P wave rate and QRS–T complex rates differ, then record these separately.

A method for the mathematician

If there is not a 6-s strip or there is a short paroxysmal tachycardia, then the heart rate can be calculated from the P–P or R–R interval as follows. At a paper speed of 25 mm/s there is 1500 mm per minute. Measure the distance, with a ruler, between two complexes (or count the number of small 1 mm boxes)

rate (in beats per minute)

$$= \frac{1500}{\text{measured distance between two complexes}}$$

At a paper speed of 50 mm/s there is 3000 mm per minute, thus:

$$\text{rate} = \frac{3000}{\text{measured distance between two complexes}}$$

2. Determine the rhythm

Check if the complexes are complete, i.e. there is a P wave for every QRS–T complex, and a QRS–T complex for every P wave.

Identifying parts of the ECG complex

In some instances it can be difficult to identify P waves, or it can be difficult to determine which are the P waves and which are the T waves (especially at fast heart rates).

Tips:
- It is often useful to mark the position of each P wave and QRS–T complex. This can be done by placing a piece of paper below the ECG tracing and placing a mark for each P and QRS (Fig. 7.1). This can help to establish if there is a pattern, or if there are hidden complexes, and if a complex has occurred before or after it was due (or expected to occur).

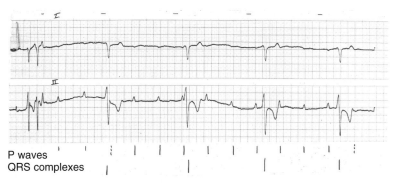

P waves
QRS complexes

Figure 7.1 ECG demonstrating how to mark out P waves and QRS complexes to help identify complexes. Note that the dotted lines represent hidden P waves – note how the first one changes the shape of the ST segment compared to others.

- Since the heart must always repolarise (to be depolarised again) there must always be a T wave following every QRS complex.
- Using callipers, note the P–R interval and Q–T interval, for a run of beats, this will often reveal which deflection must be which – as the P–R and Q–T intervals will generally remain fairly constant. This method is most usefully performed on a stretch of ECG in which there is a variation in rate.

Table 7.1 may be of assistance to the beginner – remember to always correlate the findings on auscultation of the heart and feeling the pulse with the ECG.

3. Measure the complex amplitudes and intervals

This is usually performed on a lead II rhythm strip at 50 mm/s (100 mm/s on computer print-out units) and on an unfiltered section. At 50 mm/s, 1 mm box = 0.02 seconds. Note the calibration.

Record the following (Fig. 7.2):

- P wave amplitude and duration.
- R wave amplitude and QRS duration.
- P–R interval – from start of P to start of QRS (strictly therefore a P–Q interval).
- Q–T interval – from start of QRS to end of T wave.
- Note T wave morphology.
- Note S–T segment elevation or depression.

Use the table of normal values (Table 7.2) to check if the measurements are within normal values or not.

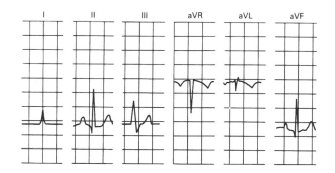

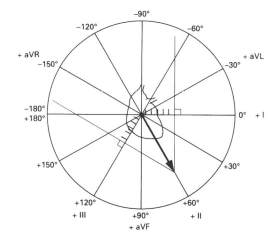

Figure 7.2 A schematic P–QRS–T complex (lead II) from a normal dog, illustrating the various amplitudes, durations and intervals (50 mm/s and 1 cm/mV).

Table 7.1 The various rhythm disturbances encountered in this book

Rhythm	Rate		ECG features			Clinical examination	
	Dog	Cat	P waves	QRS–T complexes	Additional comments	Auscultation	Pulse
Sinus rhythm	70–160	160–240	Normal	Normal		Normal	Pulse for every heart beat
Sinus arrhythmia	70–160	160–240	Normal	Normal	Rates varies Often increasing and decreasing with respiration	Normal, with variation in rate	
Sinus tachycardia	160–280	240–320	Normal	Normal		Normal but fast	
Sinus bradycardia	< 70	< 160	Normal	Normal		Normal but slow	
VPCs	–	–	None	Abnormal Occurs prematurely T wave often opposite to QRS	Overall heart rate would depend upon the frequency of the VPCs	Sounds like a tripping in the rhythm Early 'extra' beat heard with each VPC Sometimes the heart sounds with a VPC may be quiet and could sound like a 'missed' beat Very frequent VPCs can sound irregular	No pulse (or a very weak pulse) is felt with the VPC, i.e. a pulse deficit
VT	100–350	160–400	None	Abnormal QRSs Occur in sequence T wave often opposite to QRS		A sustained VT will sound normal However there will be a change in the rhythm depending upon the number of VPCs to normal beats	The pulse with a VT is usually very weak The pulse strength will vary with the frequency of the VPCs
SVPCs	–	–	Often hidden	Normal morphology Occur prematurely	If P waves are seen they are often abnormal	As for VPCs above	
SVT	160–400	240–450	Often hidden	Normal QRSs Occur in sequence R amplitude may vary slightly	If P waves are seen they are often abnormal Overall heart rate would depend upon the frequency of the SVPCs	As for VT above	
Atrial fibrillation	QRS: 100–300	QRS: 160–300	No P waves present Replaced by f waves, but f waves can be difficult to distinguish from muscle tremor	Normal QRS morphology R–R is chaotic R amplitude is variable	If there is an intraventricular conduction block, the QRS morphology will be abnormal	Chaotic rate with a variation in intensity of the heart sounds Sounds like 'shoes in a tumble dryer'	The pulse rate is often less than half the heart rate, i.e. there is > 50% pulse deficit The pulse strength is variable
Ventricular fibrillation	–	–	None	No QRS complexes evident There is a 'wavy' line which is chaotic	The heart is said to feel like a 'can of worms'	No heart sounds heard	No pulse palpable

Rhythm	Rate Dog	Rate Cat	ECG features P waves	ECG features QRS–T complexes	ECG features Additional comments	Clinical examination Auscultation	Clinical examination Pulse
Sinus block	70–160	160–240	None	None. R to R interval equals the R–R interval ×2, of the preceding normal complexes		There is a pause in the rhythm, like there has been a dropped beat	Like a missed pulse has occurred
Sinus arrest	< 160	< 240	None	None. There may be ectopic escape complexes. Pause in rhythm exceeds R–R interval ×2 of the preceding normal complexes		There is a long pause in the heart sounds	No pulse is palpated during the arrest
Atrial standstill	< 70	< 160	None	Usually abnormal, i.e. ventricular escape rhythm		Heart sounds normal, but usually slow	Pulse is palpable for each heart beat
First degree AVB	70–160	160–240	Normal	Normal		Normal	Pulse for every heart beat
Second degree AVB	P: 70–160 QRS: < 160	P: 70–160 QRS: < 240	Normal	None–intermittently	i.e. some P waves are not followed by a QRS complex	Occasional pause in heart sounds, similar to sinus block or arrest. Atrial contraction sound might be heard. If there are frequent blocked beats, the rhythm can sound irregular, but slow with pauses	No pulse felt with blocked beat
Third degree AVB	P: 70–160 QRS: < 70	P: 70–160 QRS: < 160	Normal	Normal–nodal escape or Abnormal–ventricular escape	P waves and QRS complexes are unrelated	Sounds normal, but slow, often quite a steady rate (unlike sinus arrhythmia for example). Atrial contractions sounds may be heard faintly, they are usually at a normal rate and regular	Pulse felt for each heart beat
RBBB							
LBBB	These are still normal sinus rhythms thus see rates for sinus rhythm above		Normal	Abnormal morphology but there is a P waves for every QRS		As for sinus rhythm: normal heart sounds and pulse for every beat	
LAFB							
Ventricular pre-excitation	>70	>160	Normal	Normal, except a delta wave may be seen in the upstroke of the QRS	If this leads to a supraventricular tachycardia, i.e. WPW, the rate can be 300 to 400	Normal, except when there is an SVT	Pulse every beat, but weak when there is an SVT
AV dissociation	>70	>160	Normal	Normal	Some P waves may be hidden within QRS–T complexes. There is a slight mismatch in P wave rate and QRS rate, but still almost 1:1	Most usually sounds normal	Pulse for every heart beat

This table provides guidelines, not only on the ECG characteristics, but also a guide on the heart rate at which the arrhythmias are most usually encountered (based on the author's experience) and also, but importantly, what is likely to be found on physical examination. It is important to link the ECG findings with the clinical findings and not to examine the animal one day then run an ECG on a different day, without re-examining the animal to check the clinical findings have not changed.

Abbreviations: VPCs, ventricular premature complexes; VT, ventricular tachycardia; SVPCs, supraventricular premature complexes; SVT, supraventricular tachycardia; AVB, atrioventricular block; RBBB, right bundle branch block; LBBB, left bundle branch block; LAFB, left anterior fascicular block.

Table 7.2 Guidelines on normal values for cats and dogs

		Dog	Cat
Heart rate	Adult	70–160	120–240
	Puppy	70–220	
Measurements			
P wave duration		<0.04 s	<0.04 s
	Giant breeds	<0.05 s	
P wave amplitude		<0.4 mV	<0.2 mV
P–R interval		0.06–0.13 s	0.05–0.09 s
QRS duration		<0.05 s	<0.04 s
	Giant breeds	<0.06 s	
R wave amplitudes		<2.0 mV	<0.9 mV
	Giant breeds	<2.5 mV	
S–T segment	Depression	<0.2 mV	No depression
	Elevation	<0.15 mV	No elevation
T wave		<0.25 of normal R wave amplitude	<0.3 mV
Q–T interval		0.15–0.25 s	0.12–0.18 s
Mean electrical axis		+40° to +100°	0° to +160°

4. Mean electrical axis (MEA)

This is of limited value in small animals, in part because the vector in the frontal plane (which is the plane which is measured from limb leads) is less representative of the true direction of the vector in three dimensions, compared to humans. The MEA is used mainly to assist in the assessment of ventricular enlargement and in the recognition of intraventricular conduction defects.

The value in exactly measuring the MEA in every case is questionable; a rough estimate of whether it is right or left is usually sufficient. However, the understanding on how it is measured and how it varies provides a better understanding of the 'electricity of the heart' (see Chapter 3).

How to estimate the MEA

There are a few methods to measure the MEA, two are described here. The first method was introduced earlier on page 25.

1. Eyeballing the MEA

Using this method provides a quick system and, with practice, the MEA can often be 'eyeballed' to see whether it is normal or abnormal. Look again at the diagrams in Chapter 3 describing right and left axes, and how the amplitude of the QRS complex varies in leads I, II and III with these.

Using all six limb leads and the hexaxial lead system, find the tallest (most positive) QRS complexes – the MEA is approximately in this direction. Similarly, find the most negative complexes, the MEA is opposite in direction to this. Alternatively, find the lead in which the QRS complex is equally positive and negative (and usually small) – this is called the isoelectric lead. The MEA will be perpendicular to this. Find which of the six limb leads is perpendicular to the isoelectric lead. If the perpendicular lead is positive, then the MEA is in that direction. If the perpendicular lead is negative, then the MEA is in the opposite direction to that lead.

2. Triangulation

Using two leads from a good quality tracing, commonly leads I and III are used, but in fact any two leads can be used, measure the net amplitude of the QRS complex in each lead. In other words, measure the amplitude of the QRS complex that is positive and the amplitude that is negative. Subtract one (the smaller) from the other – this is the net amplitude. Plot this, to scale, on the hexaxial lead system shown below (Fig. 7.3). Draw perpendicular lines from each point. Where the two lines meet is the direction of the MEA from the centre point.

In fact, if the net amplitude in all six leads is calculated and plotted on the hexaxial lead system, the lines that are drawn perpendicular from each point should all meet at approximately the same point.

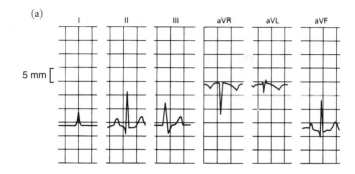

(a)

5 mm

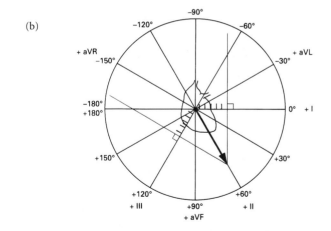

(b)

Figure 7.3 Estimation of mean electrical axis. (a) *Method 1*. In this normal canine ECG, lead aVL is the most isoelectric lead. Perpendicular to this is lead II. Lead II is positive and therefore the MEA is towards the positive pole of this line, i.e. +60°. (b) *Method 2*. In the same ECG. The net amplitude in lead I is +6 (Q = 0 and R = +6). Plot 6 points along lead I in the hexaxial lead system diagram and draw a perpendicular. The net amplitude in lead III is +6 (S = −2 and R = +8). Plot 6 points along lead III and draw a perpendicular. Draw an arrow from the centre to where the two perpendicular lines intersect. This is the direction of the MEA, i.e. +60°.

PART 3
Abnormalities of the ECG complex and abnormal rhythms

8 • Changes in the P–QRS–T morphology

Wandering pacemaker

This occurs as a result of the dominant pacemaker shifting from the SA node to other pacemaker cells with a high intrinsic rate within the atria. Sometimes referred to as a wandering atrial pacemaker.

ECG characteristics

P waves can vary in morphology, i.e. there is a variation in amplitude.

The P waves can vary from positive, negative or biphasic, or even be isoelectric and be so small that they are difficult to identify (Fig. 8.1).

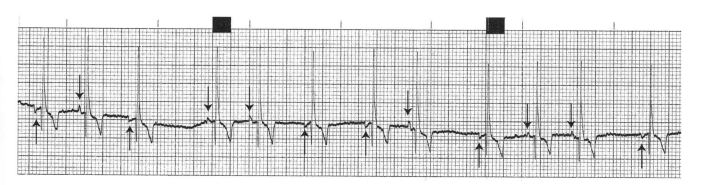

Figure 8.1 ECG from a dog showing a wandering pacemaker. Note how the P wave morphology changes (arrows) – this is not an abnormality in dogs (lead II, 25 mm/s and 1 cm/mV).

Clinical significance

This is normal, and not uncommon in dogs, and is thought to be associated with high vagal tone. Its significance is therefore similar to sinus arrhythmia (see pages 12 and 13).

Changes associated with chamber enlargement

The ECG should not be viewed as being a means to diagnose heart enlargement in small animals, but as an additional diagnostic test that might help to support such a clinical suspicion. Chest radiographs are often considered a more reliable indicator of heart enlargement. Echocardiography is probably the best means to assess chamber size and morphology.

Note that in 'ECG-speak', 'enlargement' is commonly used to encompass either hypertrophy or dilation, as these can rarely be distinguished reliably on an ECG.

Table 7.2 lists normal values giving ECG complex durations and amplitudes. Measurements are usually measured in lead II at 50 mm/s, unfiltered.

Left atrial enlargement

When there is left atrial (LA) enlargement (or dilation) the P wave is often prolonged and sometimes also notched (Fig. 8.2). A prolonged and notched P wave is referred to as **P-mitrale** (as LA enlargement is often associated with mitral valve disease). The notching occurs as a result of asynchronous depolarisation of the atria, the dilated left atrium depolarising

fractionally later then the right atrium. *Note*: giant breeds often normally have slightly prolonged P waves.

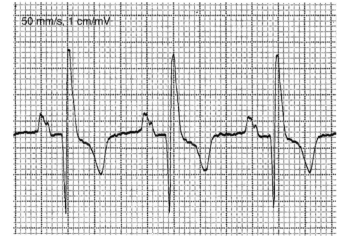

Figure 8.2 ECG illustrating prolonged (0.6 s) and notched P waves, this is termed P-mitrale. From an 8-year-old Dobermann with dilated cardiomyopathy.

Right atrial enlargement

When there is right atrial (RA) enlargement (or dilation) the P wave is increased in amplitude (Fig. 8.3). Such tall P waves are referred to as **P-pulmonale** (as RA enlargement may be associated with cor pulmonale). Note that P-pulmonale is commonly seen in breeds which are predisposed to chronic airway disease.

Left ventricular enlargement

Tall R waves are suggestive of left ventricular (LV) enlargement (Fig. 8.4). An R wave in lead I greater than leads II or aVF, may be associated with hypertrophy. An increased in R waves in leads I, II and III may be associated with dilation. Other ECG features that may be associated with LV enlargement are: prolongation of the QRS duration, S–T segment sagging/coving (see page 72) or a shift in the MEA to the left.

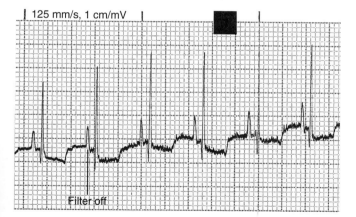

Figure 8.3 ECG illustrating tall P waves (0.5 mV), this is termed P-pulmonale. There is fine muscle tremor artifact affecting the baseline. From a 10-year-old Yorkshire terrier with long-standing tracheal collapse.

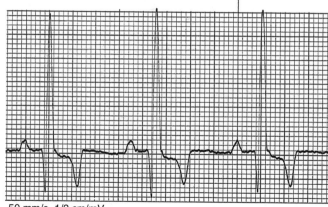

Figure 8.4 ECG illustrating tall R waves (6.0 mV) and prolonged QRS complex duration (0.06 s) which is suggestive of left ventricular enlargement. From a 1-year-old German Shepherd dog with a patent ductus arteriosus.

Right ventricular enlargement

Deep S waves are suggestive of right ventricular (RV) enlargement (Fig. 8.5). Other ECG features that may be associated with RV enlargement are: prolongation of the QRS duration or a shift in the MEA to the right.

Abnormal mean electrical axis (MEA)

A **right axis** may suggest right ventricular enlargement (Fig. 8.5), but may be due to displacement of the heart within the chest to the right side or might even be a normal-variation. A conduction disturbance such as right bundle branch block (see page 102) also produces a right axis deviation.

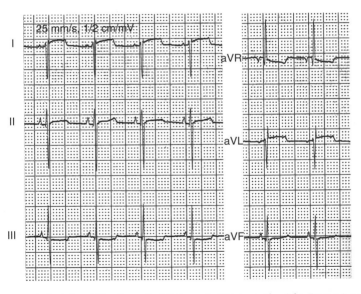

Figure 8.5 ECG illustrating deep S waves in leads I and II and an axis shift towards aVR, i.e. to the right. From a 2-year-old West Highland white terrier with pulmonic stenosis.

A **left axis** may be due to left ventricular enlargement, but may be due to displacement of the heart within the chest to the left or it may be a normal-variation. A conduction disturbance such as left anterior fascicular block (see page 104) also produces a left axis deviation.

Low-voltage QRS complexes

QRS complexes will be smaller the further the electrodes are from the heart and depending on the resistance to electrical conduction between the heart and the electrodes. For example, the ECG complexes are larger in precordial chest leads, which are very close to the heart. However, complexes can be small in limb leads in obese animals. Heavy filtering on the

ECG machine can also reduce the amplitude of the ECG complexes significantly.

ECG characteristics

An R wave amplitude less than 0.5 mV in the limb leads is considered small in dogs (Fig. 8.6). QRS complexes are usually small in normal cats.

Clinical significance

Small complexes in dogs may be due to obesity, effusions (pericardial, pleural, ascites), hypothyroidism, hyperkalaemia,

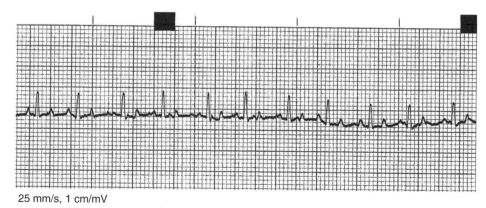

25 mm/s, 1 cm/mV

Figure 8.6 ECG illustrating small ECG complexes in a dog.

pneumothorax, some respiratory diseases, hypovolaemia or it may be a normal-variation.

Electrical alternans

ECG characteristics

This is an alternation in QRS amplitude that occurs nearly every other beat (Fig. 8.7).

Clinical significance

Electrical alternans is associated with movement of the heart within pericardial effusion, which is evident on echocardio-graphy where the heart can be seen to 'bounce' from side to side within pericardial fluid as it beats. This movement of the heart causes a slight alternating change in the cardiac axis and is seen on the ECG as an alternating variation in QRS amplitude. Note that this should not be confused with the more gradual variation in amplitude seen with respiration in some animals, nor the variation seen with a supraventricular tachycardia or atrial fibrillation.

Notching in the R wave

Although these abnormalities can be seen commonly in heart disease in small animals, the significance of notches is debat-

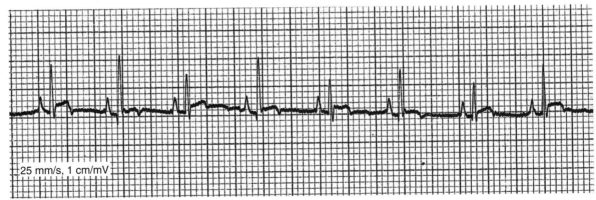

25 mm/s, 1 cm/mV

Figure 8.7 ECG illustrating electrical alternans – note the alternating amplitude of the R waves. From a Golden Retriever with pericardial effusion due to idiopathic pericarditis.

able – it is the 'heart disease' that is of greater importance than trying to analyse every minutiae. Notches in the QRS complex are reported to occur with microscopic intramural myocardial infarction or associated with areas of myocardial fibrosis (Fig. 8.8). Notches in the QRS complex are also seen with intra-ventricular conduction defects (see page 101) and a slight notch is sometimes also seen with ventricular pre-excitation in the upstroke of the R wave (see page 104). Notches can also be produced artifactually in tracings in which there is excessive muscle tremor or electrical interference.

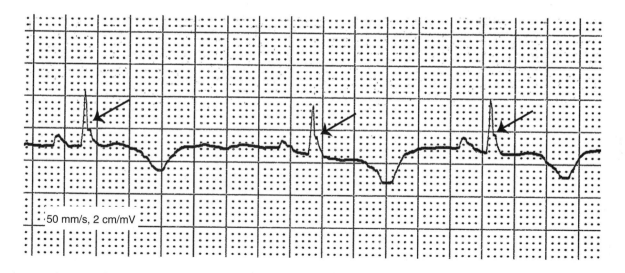

50 mm/s, 2 cm/mV

Figure 8.8 ECG illustrating notching in the QRS complex. From a cat with dilated cardiomyopathy.

Q–T interval abnormalities

The Q–T interval varies a little, inversely with heart rate, so it is difficult to accurately define what is exactly abnormal.

Clinical significance

Prolonged Q–T intervals may be seen in:

- hypocalcaemia
- hypokalaemia
- hypothermia
- quinidine
- ethylene glycol poisoning.

Shortened Q–T interval may be seen in:

- hyperkalaemia
- hypercalcaemia
- digitalis
- atropine
- beta-blockers and calcium channel antagonists.

S–T segment abnormalities

S–T elevation is seen in:

- pericarditis
- severe ischaemia/infarction, e.g. full wall thickness.

S–T depression is seen in (Fig. 8.9):

- endomyocardial ischaemia (e.g. cardiomyopathy, trauma)
- potassium imbalance
- digitalis toxicity.

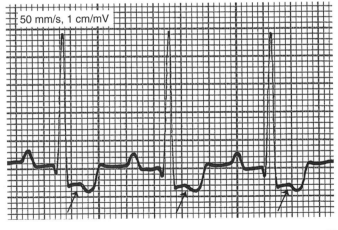

50 mm/s, 1 cm/mV

Figure 8.9 ECG illustrating depression of the S–T segment. From a 4-year-old Staffordshire Bull Terrier with mitral valve dysplasia.

Abnormalities of the T wave

The morphology of T waves in small animal is very variable and the diagnostic value of T wave changes is very limited compared to humans. A higher value might be placed on T wave changes compared to a previous recording in the same animal. The most common abnormal change is the development of large T waves (Fig. 8.10). This can be associated with hyperkalaemia (see below) or myocardial hypoxia.

Hyperkalaemia

Hyperkalaemia is a well known cause of ECG abnormalities (Fig. 8.10), but it must be remembered that a normal ECG would not exclude hyperkalaemia (or Addison's disease) and serum electrolytes levels should always be measured (and an adrenocorticotrophic test performed) if this is suspected.

ECG characteristics

The ECG changes vary with increasing severity of the hyperkalaemia as follows:

- there is a progressive bradycardia
- increased amplitude of the T wave, appearing narrow and spiked
- progressive decrease in amplitude of the R wave
- progressive reduction in amplitude of the P wave
- disappearance of the P wave, i.e. atrial standstill, with a slow junctional (nodal) rhythm
- finally ventricular fibrillation or asystole.

Clinical significance

Hyperkalaemia may be associated with Addison's disease, acute renal shutdown (e.g. feline urethral obstruction syndrome), diabetic ketoacidosis and severe skeletal muscle damage.

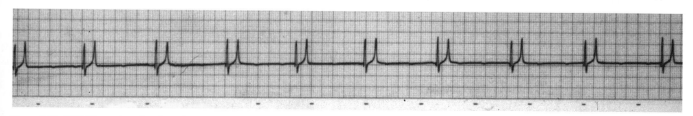

Figure 8.10 ECG illustrating a bradycardia at 50/min, the absence of P waves (atrial standstill) and tall peaked T waves from a dog with hyperkalaemia (25 mm/s and 1 cm/mV).

9 • Abnormalities associated with ectopia

'Ectopia' literally means 'in an abnormal place'. In reference to the heart this means outwith the SA node, the dominant pacemaker. Ectopic beats arise as a result of various mechanisms due to a number of causes (e.g. cardiac pathology, hypoxia, electrolyte imbalances).

Terminology

The electrocardiographic interpretation of dysrhythmias due to ectopia requires an understanding of the terminology used. If this is accomplished, interpretation becomes relatively easy. It might also be useful, at this point, to review Chapter 3 (Abnormal electricity of the heart).

The term 'beat' implies that there has been an actual contraction. In 'ECG-speak' it is better to use the term **complex** or **depolarisation** to describe waveforms on the electrocardiograph.

Ectopic complexes may be classified by the following:

1. *Site of origin* (Fig. 9.1). They are either ventricular or

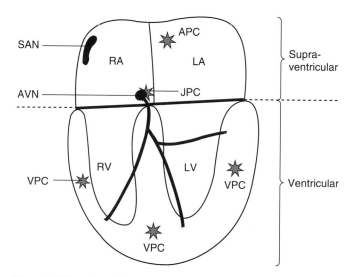

Figure 9.1 Illustration of the origin of supraventricular and ventricular ectopic complexes. SAN – sinoatrial node; AVN – atrioventricular node; APC – atrial premature complex; JPC – junctional premature complex; VPC – ventricular premature complex; RA – right atrium; LA – left atrium; RV – right ventricle; LV – left ventricle.

supraventricular. Supraventricular ectopics may be sub-classified into either: (a) atrial (originating in the atria) or (b) junctional or nodal (originating in the AV node or bundle of His).

2. *Timing.* Ectopic complexes that occur before the next normal complex would have been due are termed **premature**, and those that occur following a pause such as a period of sinus arrest or in complete heart block are termed **escape** complexes (Fig. 9.2).

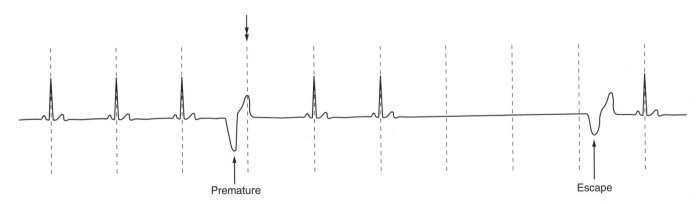

Premature   Escape

Figure 9.2 Illustration of (1) a ventricular premature complex (the double-headed arrow indicates the timing of when the next normal sinus complex would have occurred) and (2) a ventricular escape beat which occurred following a pause in the rhythm.

3. *Morphology.* If all the ectopics in a tracing have a similar morphology to each other they are referred to as **uniform** and those in which there are different shapes as **multiform** (Fig. 9.3).

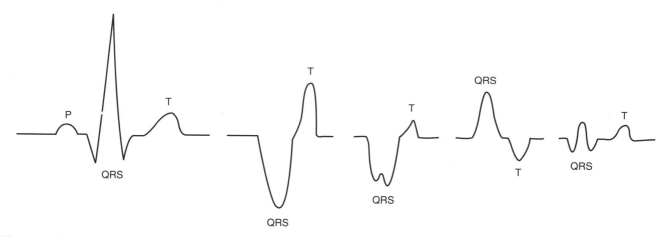

Figure 9.3 Illustration of a normal complex (first complex), followed by four examples of QRS–T complexes with an abnormal morphology due to ventricular ectopic depolarisations. It is paramount to identify the morphology of the QRS complex associated with a sinus complex (first complex). Any QRS complexes of a different morphology (for that animal) must arise from an ectopic ventricular focus.

4. *Number of ectopics.* Premature ectopic complexes may occur singly, in pairs (Fig. 9.4) or in runs of three or more; the latter is referred to as a **tachycardia**. A tachycardia may be continuous, termed **persistent** or **sustained**, or intermittent, termed **paroxysmal**.

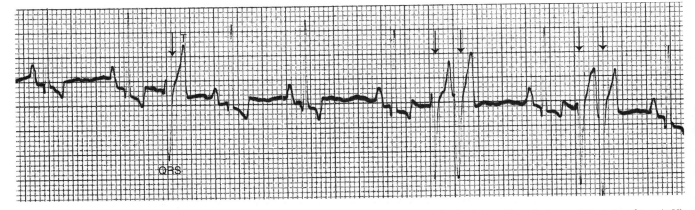

Figure 9.4 ECG with ventricular premature complexes (arrows), singly and in pairs. From a German Shepherd dog with a splenic mass (25 mm/s and 1 cm/mV).

5. *Frequency*. The number of premature ectopic complexes in a tracing may vary from occasional to very frequent. When there is a set ratio such as one sinus complex to one ectopic complex it is termed **bigeminy** (Fig. 9.5) and one ectopic to two sinus complexes is termed **trigeminy**.

Ventricular premature complexes

Ventricular premature complexes (VPCs) are a common find-ing in dogs and cats. VPCs arise from an ectopic focus or foci within the ventricular myocardium. Depolarisation therefore occurs in an abnormal direction through the myocardium and the impulse conducts from cell to cell (not within the conduction tissue).

ECG characteristics

The QRS complex morphology is abnormal, i.e. *unlike* a QRS

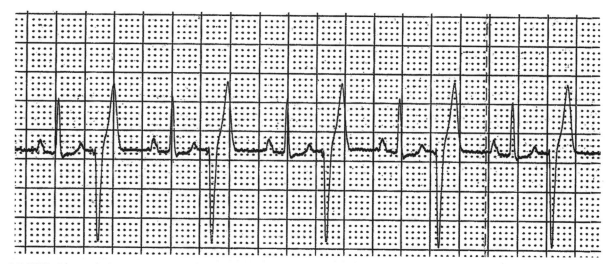

Figure 9.5 ECG with ventricular premature complexes that alternate with normal sinus complexes, this is termed ventricular bigeminy. From a 13-year-old Standard Poodle with mitral valve disease (25 mm/s and 0.5 cm/mV).

that would have arisen via the AV node (Fig. 9.6a, b). It is usually:

- abnormal (bizarre) in shape
- usually wide (prolonged)
- the T wave of a VPC is often large and opposite in direction to the QRS.

Since a VPC occurs prematurely, a normal sinus depolarisation arriving at the AV node will meet ventricles which are refractory, with its P wave usually hidden by the ventricular premature complex.

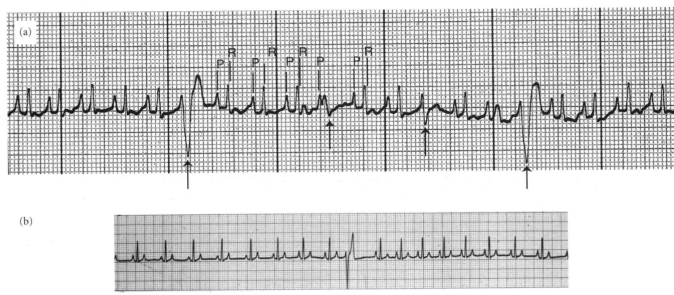

Figure 9.6 (a) ECG from a cat with multiform ventricular premature complexes (VPCs) – arrowed. Note the different morphology of the second VPC, this may be a combination of a normal QRS complex and a VPC – this is termed a fusion complex. From a 6-year-old domestic short-haired cat with hypertrophic cardiomyopathy (25 mm/s and 2 cm/mV). (b) ECG from a 10-year-old Labrador dog with a single ventricular premature complex (VPC). Note the abnormal QRS-T morphology and the premature timing (25 mm/s and 1 cm/mV).

When a VPC is so premature that it is superimposed on the T wave of the preceding complex (sinus or ectopic), i.e. the ventricles are depolarised before they have completely repolarised from the preceding contraction, this is termed **R-on-T** (Fig. 9.7).

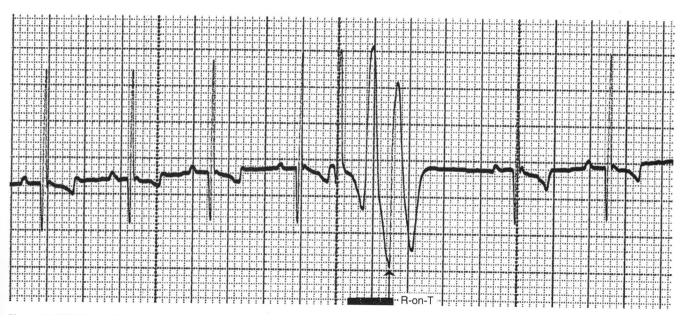

R-on-T

Figure 9.7 ECG from a dog showing a two ventricular premature complex (VPC) occurring very quickly, such that the QRS complex of the second is virtually superimposed on the T wave of the previous VPC (arrowed) – this is termed R on T (25 mm/s and 1 cm/mV).

A run of three or more VPCs is termed a **ventricular tachycardia** (Fig. 9.8).

Clinical significance

Infrequent VPCs do not generally compromise the cardiac output and, therefore, often do not require treatment (although treatment should be directed towards the underlying cause).

However, with a rapid VT there is a marked reduction in cardiac output and animals may present with exercise intolerance, lethargy or collapse. VPCs may occur due to:

- primary heart disease such as cardiac neoplasia, cardiomyopathy (particularly in Dobermanns and Boxers), myocarditis (e.g. traumatic myocarditis/contusion), endocarditis or
- secondary to a systemic disorder such as gastric dilation,

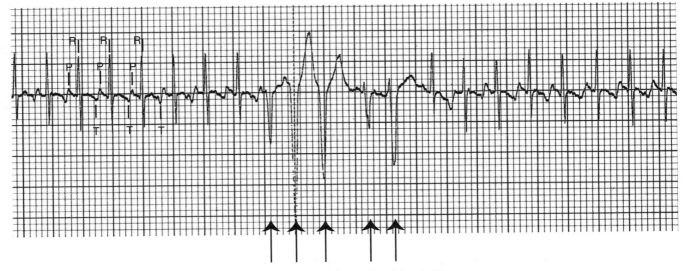

Figure 9.8 (a) ECG showing a paroxysmal ventricular tachycardia (arrows) (25 mm/s and 1 cm/mV).

pancreatitis, splenic masses, electrolyte imbalance, uraemia, pyometra and low blood oxygen saturation (e.g. hypoxia associated with congestive heart failure or respiratory diseases). Drugs such as digitalis, anaesthetics, atropine and isoprenaline may also produce VPCs.

VT, multiform VPCs and ventricular bigeminy are usually associated with severe underlying heart disease or a systemic disorder. R-on-T is believed to lead potentially to the development of ventricular fibrillation and sudden death. Therefore it is considered an important finding that would warrant management of the associated ectopia.

Supraventricular premature complexes

Supraventricular premature complexes (SVPCs) arise from an ectopic focus or foci above the ventricles, i.e. in either the atria, the AV node or bundle of His. The ventricles are then depolarised normally producing a normal-shaped QRS complex with a normal duration. Although SVPCs can be classified further into either atrial premature complexes or junctional (nodal) premature complexes, the description of these are outside the intended coverage of this book.

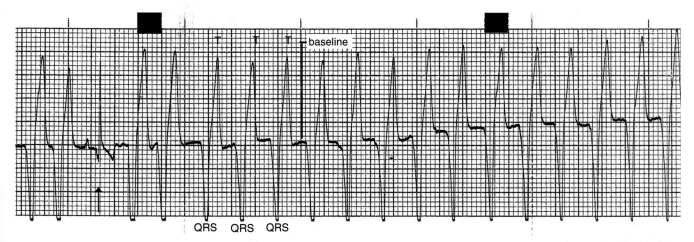

Figure 9.8 (b) ECG showing a ventricular tachycardia (VT) at 200/min. There is one normal sinus complex (arrowed). From a 10-year-old Labrador with liver neoplasia (25 mm/s and 1 cm/mV).

ECG characteristics

QRS–T complexes, which have a *normal* morphology, are seen to occur prematurely (Fig. 9.9). The ECG features are:

- normal QRS morphology (except with bundle branch block – see page 101)
- QRS seen to occur prematurely
- P waves may or may not be identified
- if P waves are seen, they are usually of an abnormal morphology (i.e. non-sinus) and the P–R interval will differ from a normal sinus complex.

A run of three or more SVPCs is termed a **supraventricular tachycardia (SVT)**, it is usually at a rate in excess of 160 per min (but can be as high as 400/min) and regular (Fig. 9.10). SVT needs to be distinguished from a sinus tachycardia.

Clinical significance

Infrequent SVPCs do not generally compromise the cardiac output and therefore often do not require treatment (although treatment should be directed towards the underlying cause). However, with a rapid SVT there is a marked reduction in cardiac output and animals may present with exercise intolerance, lethargy, episodic weakness or recumbency.

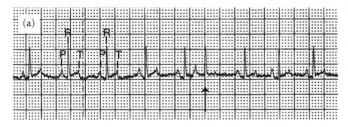

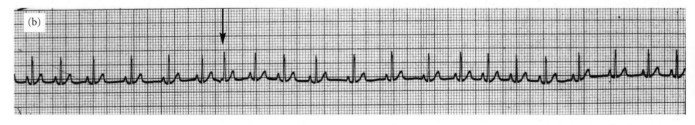

Figure 9.9 (a) ECG showing a single supraventricular premature complex (arrowed). Note the premature timing and absence of an obvious P wave. An incidental finding from a 9-year-old Newfoundland dog (25 mm/s and 1 cm/mV). (b) ECG from a dog. Note the premature complex (arrowed) with a normal QRS-T morphology – this is a supraventricular premature complex (SVPC) (25 mm/s and 1 cm/mV).

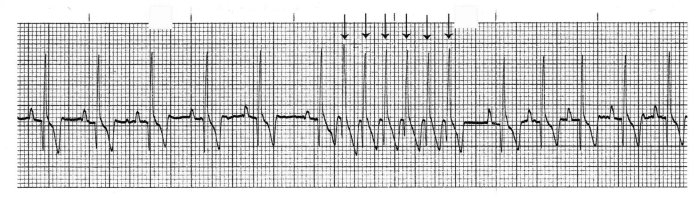

Figure 9.10 (a) ECG showing a paroxysmal supraventricular tachycardia (arrowed) (25 mm/s and 1 cm/mV).

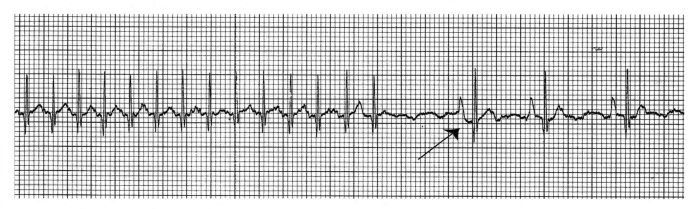

Figure 9.10 (b) ECG showing initially a supraventricular tachycardia at 280/min which then breaks to a normal sinus rhythm at 90/min (the first sinus complex is arrowed). From a 6-year-old Irish Wolfhound with occult dilated cardiomyopathy (25 mm/s and 1 cm/mV).

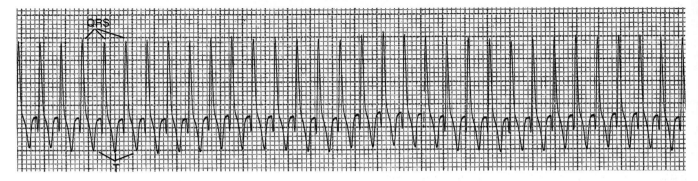

Figure 9.10 (c) ECG showing a sustained supraventricular tachycardia at 320/min. From a 9-year-old Weimaraner with myocarditis (25 mm/s and 0.5 cm/mV).

SVPCs can be due to:

- atrial disease, e.g. dilation/stretch secondary to AV valve regurgitation (associated with congenital and acquired AV valve disease, cardiomyopathy, congenital cardiac shunts), right atrial haemangiosarcoma or
- secondary to some systemic illness including hyperthyroidism in cats, or a side-effect of some drugs, e.g. digitalis toxicity or 'stimulant'-type drugs.

Escape rhythms

When the dominant pacemaker tissue (usually the SA node) fails to discharge for a long period, pacemaker tissue with a slower intrinsic rate (junctional or ventricular) may then discharge, i.e. they 'escape' the control of the SA node. This is commonly seen in association with bradydysrhythmias (e.g. sinus bradycardia, sinus arrest, AV block). Escape complexes are sometimes referred to as rescue beats, because if they did not occur death would be imminent.

If no escape rhythm developed, i.e. there was no electrical activity of any kind, then this is termed **asystole**. It would not be dissimilar to sustained sinus arrest if no escape rhythm developed. This is a terminal event unless electrical activity returns. If there is a failure of an escape rhythm during complete heart block, i.e. there are P waves but no QRS complexes, then this is termed **ventricular standstill**. Again, if ventricular electrical activity does not return death is imminent.

Junctional escapes are fairly normal in shape (i.e. junctional ectopic), whereas ventricular escapes are abnormal and bizarre (i.e. ventricular ectopic) see Figs 9.11 and 10.2. A continuous junctional escape rhythm occurs at a rate of 60–70 per min and a continuous ventricular escape rhythm occurs at a rate of less than 50 per min. Either may be seen in complete AV block.

Clinical significance

Since they are rescue beats they should not be suppressed by any form of treatment. Treatment should be directed towards the underlying bradydysrhythmia.

AV dissociation

AV dissociation describes the situation when the atria and ventricles are depolarised by separate independent foci. This may occur due to an accelerated junctional or ventricular rhythm, disturbed AV conduction or depressed SA nodal function.

ECG characteristics

The ECG shows a ventricular rate that is usually very slightly faster than the atrial rate. The P waves may occur before, during or after the QRS complex. The P waves and QRS complexes are independent of each other with the QRS complexes appear-

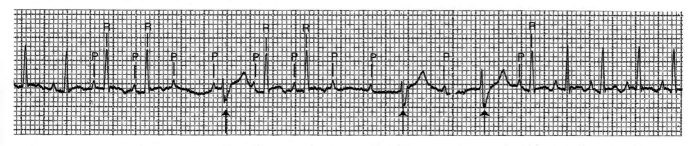

Figure 9.11 ECG from a 7-year-old cat with intermittent failure of AV nodal conduction through to the ventricles (non-conducted P waves), i.e. second degree heart block (see later). Following the consequential pauses in ventricular depolarisation, ventricular escape complexes occur (arrowed) (25 mm/s and 2 cm/mV).

ing to 'catch up' on the P waves (Fig. 9.12). Complete AV block is one form of AV dissociation, but AV dissociation does not mean there is AV block.

Clinical significance

AV dissociation is commonly seen in cats during anaesthesia and in animals with cardiomyopathy or electrolyte disturbances. It is not a haemodynamically significant arrhythmia, but the cause of the AV dissociation should be treated (see supraventricular and ventricular tachycardia).

Fibrillation

Fibrillation means rapid irregular small movements of fibres.

Atrial fibrillation

This is probably one of the most common arrhythmias seen in small animals. On auscultation the heart sounds rapid and randomly irregular, and the pulse rate is often half the heart rate. In atrial fibrillation (AF) depolarisation waves occur randomly throughout the atria. Since AF originates above the

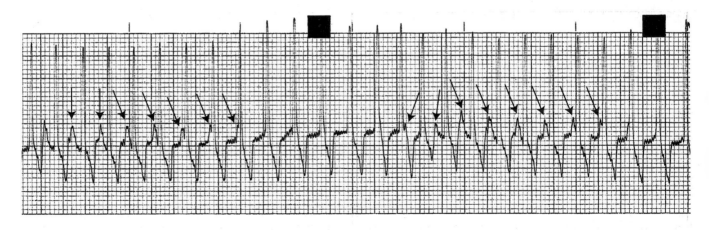

Figure 9.12 ECG showing AV dissociation. Note how the P waves (arrows) appear to drift in and out of the QRS complexes (the P–R interval is variable in AV dissociation). Incidental finding from a 13-year-old Samoyed dog (25 mm/s and 1 cm/mV).

ventricles, it could also be classified as a supraventricular arrhythmia.

ECG characteristics

The QRS complexes have a normal morphology (similar to supraventricular premature complexes described previously) and occur at a normal to fast rate (Fig. 9.13). The ECG features are:

- normal QRS morphology (except when there is bundle branch block – see page 101)

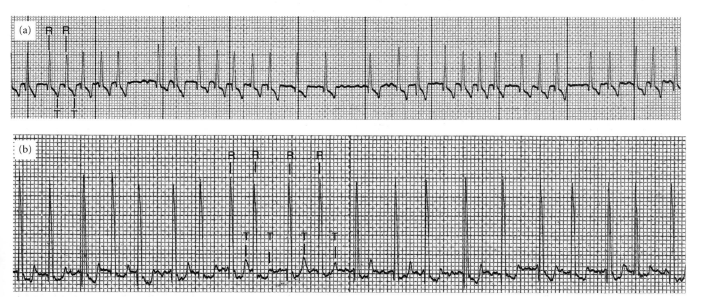

Figure 9.13 (a) ECG showing atrial fibrillation with an average ventricular response rate of 180/min. The QRS complexes are chaotic – this is usually easier to hear on auscultation of the heart. There are no P waves discernible, although the fine undulations of the baseline may be flutter waves in this instance (25 mm/s and 1 cm/mV). (b) ECG showing atrial fibrillation with an average ventricular response rate of 180/min. There is some baseline interference due to muscle tremor artifact – note how this masks identification of flutter waves. From a 5-year-old Mastiff dog with dilated cardiomyopathy (25 mm/s and 1 cm/mV).

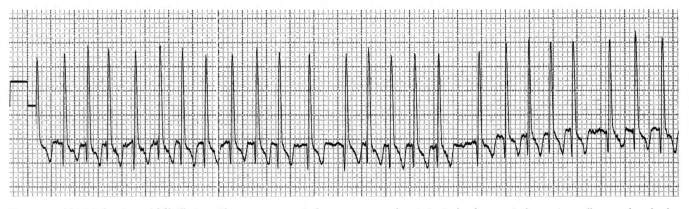

Figure 9.13 (c) ECG showing atrial fibrillation with an average ventricular response rate of 280/min. Such a fast ventricular rate is usually seen when the dog is in congestive heart failure. From a 7-year-old Dobermann with pulmonary oedema due to dilated cardiomyopathy (25 mm/s and 0.5 cm/mV).

- R–R interval is irregular and chaotic (this is easier to hear on auscultation!)
- the QRS complexes often vary in amplitude
- there are no recognisable P waves preceding the QRS complex
- sometimes fine irregular movements of the baseline are seen as a result of the atrial fibrillation waves – referred to as 'f' **waves**, however these are frequently indistinguishable from baseline artefact (e.g. muscle tremor) in small animals.

Clinical significance

Atrial fibrillation usually occurs as a result of dilation and stretching of one or both atria and is most commonly seen in medium- to large-breed dogs with dilated cardiomyopathy. However, it can occur in any breed of dog associated with atrial stretch secondary to AV valve incompetence, congenital cardiac shunts, heart base tumours and sometimes following rapid drainage of a pericardial effusion. It is uncommon in the cat, but is sometimes seen when there is severe left atrial dilation secondary to hypertrophic cardiomyopathy. Atrial fibrillation does not have major haemodynamic affects. The loss of the atrial contraction contribution to cardiac output is approximately 10–20%, which is compensated for primarily by an increase in rate. Atrial fibrillation is sometimes seen in giant-breed dogs with no gross cardiac pathology – referred to as 'lone' AF. Lone AF usually has a fairly normal ventricular rate, as there is no increase in sympathetic drive since the dogs are not in heart failure. However, many giant-breed dogs with lone AF progress to dilated cardiomyopathy and ultimately heart failure.

Ventricular fibrillation (VF)

This is nearly always a terminal event associated with cardiac arrest. The depolarisation waves occur randomly throughout the ventricles. There is therefore no significant co-ordinated contraction to produce any cardiac output. If the heart is visualised or palpated, fine irregular movements of the ventricles are evident – likened to a 'can of worms'. VF can often follow ventricular tachycardia.

ECG characteristics

The ECG shows **coarse** (larger) or **fine** (smaller) rapid, irregular and bizarre movement with no normal wave or complex (Fig. 9.14).

Clinical significance

Death usually ensues unless rapid cardiopulmonary resuscitation is initiated with electrical defibrillation. However, the success of this will depend on the extent of existing pathology. The causes are numerous, but not dissimilar to those of VPCs and VT.

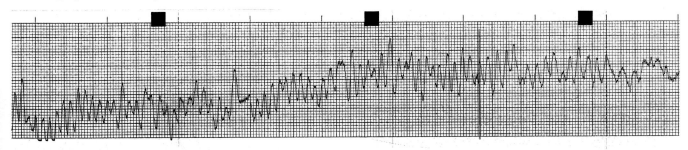

Figure 9.14 ECG showing ventricular flutter/fibrillation. From an 11-year-old German Shepherd dog that died on arrival with advanced cardiac tamponade due to pericardial haemorrhage (25 mm/s and 1 cm/mV).

10 • Abnormalities in the conduction system

Abnormalities in the conduction system are associated with faults in either the generation of the impulse from the SA node or abnormalities in conduction through the specialised conduction tissue, i.e. the AV node, bundle of His and Purkinje system.

Sinus arrest and block

When there is a failure of the SA node to generate an impulse, i.e. the SA node has temporarily arrested – it is referred to as **sinus arrest**. However, if it is a failure of the impulse to be conducted from the SA node to the atrial muscle, i.e. the impulse is blocked from depolarising the atria. This is referred to as **sinus block**.

ECG characteristics

There is a pause in the rhythm with neither a P wave nor a QRS–T complex, i.e. the baseline is flat (except for movement artifact if present). If the pause is only twice the R–R interval, it suggests sinus block. However, if the pause is greater than two R–R intervals, it suggests sinus arrest (Fig. 10.1). Long

periods of arrest are often followed by ventricular ectopic escape complexes.

Clinical significance

A long period of sinus arrest may result in **syncope**, as no blood flows to the brain and fainting occurs. How long the period

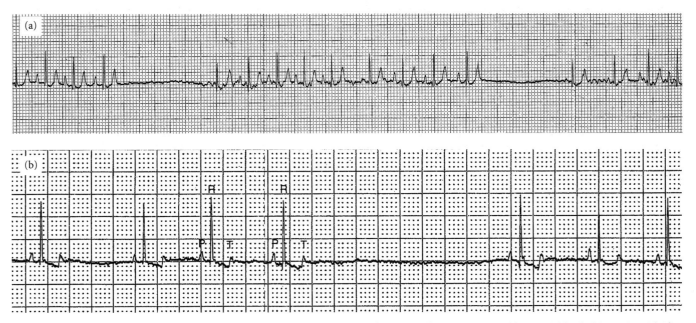

Figure 10.1 (a) ECG showing a intermittent sinus arrest – the pauses are approximately 1.5 seconds. From a 9-year-old West Highland white terrier with idiopathic pulmonary fibrosis (25 mm/s and 1 cm/mV). (b) ECG from a Lakeland terrier with sinus arrest – there is a 2-second pause (25 mm/s and 1 cm/mV).

of sinus arrest must be to result in syncope depends on the activity (or metabolic rate) of the animal, e.g. a 5-second pause may be sufficient when running, but it may require 15–25 seconds at rest. **Pre-syncope** occurs if the duration of the sinus arrest is not quite sufficient to result in collapse but does cause signs of weakness or stumbling.

Sinus arrest/block can be a normal finding in some brachycephalic dogs when it is considered to be an exaggerated respiratory sinus arrhythmia.

There are several conditions that may be associated with sinus arrest that overlap with causes of sinus bradycardia (see pages 14 and 15):

- It may be one feature of sick sinus syndrome.
- Vagal stimulation associated with severe respiratory disease (it can be normal in dogs with brachycephalic upper airway syndrome for example) or associated with a vasovagal response, e.g. with vomiting or tenesmus.
- Atrial disease such as dilation, fibrosis, cardiomyopathy or neoplasia (e.g. haemangiosarcoma and heart base tumours).
- Metabolic or endocrine diseases such as an electrolyte imbalance or hypothyroidism.
- Drugs either due to their effects or associated with toxicity must also be considered.
- Irritation of the vagus nerve by neoplasia in the cervical area (e.g. thyroid carcinoma) or in the thorax (e.g. aortic body tumour). Surgical manipulation within the thorax may also result in sinus arrest.

Sick-sinus syndrome

This is a term for an abnormally functioning SA node and is probably better termed **sinus node dysfunction**. This 'umbrella' term refers to any abnormality of sinus node function including severe sinus bradycardia and severe sinus arrest. In some situations the profound bradycardia alternates with a supraventricular tachycardia (Fig. 10.2), this is termed the **'bradycardia–tachycardia syndrome'**. Sick sinus syndrome has

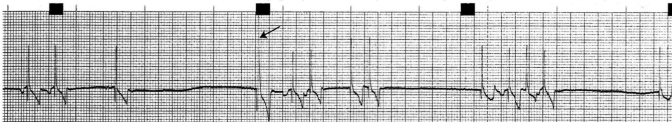

Figure 10.2 ECG from a 10-year-old miniature Schnauzer with sick sinus syndrome. This tracing shows periods of sinus arrest alternating with supraventricular premature complexes. There is one ventricular escape present (arrowed) (25 mm/s and 1 cm/mV).

been reported to occur most commonly in female miniature Schnauzers at least 6 years of age. It has not been recorded in cats.

ECG characteristics

The electrocardiographic features are therefore quite variable and include persisting sinus bradycardia or episodes of sinus arrest without escape beats. One feature of sick sinus syndrome is that during long periods of sinus arrest there is often a failure of rescue escape beats. In the bradycardia–tachycardia syndrome there are periods of bradycardia such as sinus arrest, alternating with a supraventricular tachycardia. The bradycardia may be unresponsive to an injection of atropine.

Clinical significance

As for sinus arrest described previously, prolonged periods of no cardiac output will result in pre-syncope or syncope. A profound sinus bradycardia may present with lethargy and exercise intolerance due to an inability to increase cardiac output on demand. In the bradycardia–tachycardia syndrome either the bradycardia or the tachycardia may produce a significant drop in cardiac output and result in weakness or syncope.

The treatment of choice for symptomatic cases is pacemaker implantation and possibly also the addition of antidysrhyth-mic drugs. It is usually difficult to obtain satisfactory rate control with medical treatment alone.

Atrial standstill

In atrial standstill there is an absence of any atrial activity, which can be confirmed by fluoroscopy or echocardiography. This occurs due to a failure of atrial muscle depolarisation, i.e. the SA node may produce an impulse, but the atria are not depolarised and remain inactive. The impulses are conducted from the SA node by internodal pathways to the AV node. Thus there is a nodal (or junctional) escape rhythm in these cases. The escape rhythm is called a sinoventricular rhythm.

ECG characteristics

The electrocardiographic feature is of the absence of P waves usually with a slow (less than 60 per min) escape rhythm (Fig. 10.3). The quality of the ECG has to be excellent (i.e. the baseline must be flat without any artifacts) to confidently diagnose the absence of P waves. The QRS complexes are often of a relatively normal shape (junctional escape), but sometimes with a slightly prolonged duration. In a few cases the escape rhythm can be ventricular.

Clinical significance

Atrial standstill can be classified in to three types, based on the underlying condition.

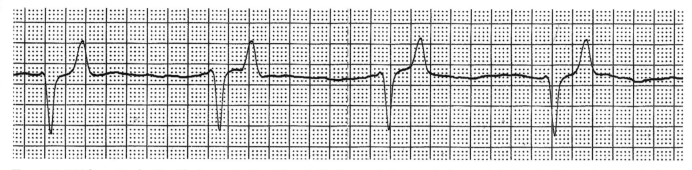

Figure 10.3 ECG from a Cavalier King Charles spaniel with atrial standstill with a ventricular escape rhythm at 70/min. Note the absence of P waves. The absence of atrial activity can be confirmed by echocardiography (50 mm/s and 1 cm/mV).

- One type has been reported in English springer spaniels, old English sheep dogs and mixed breed dogs and the author has seen cases in cavalier king Charles spaniels. This type is referred to as **persistent** atrial standstill and is poorly responsive to any medication, including atropine, or even pacemaker implantation (in the author's experience). The clinical signs are usually of weakness, lethargy and syncope associated with the reduction in cardiac output and inability to increase the heart rate during activity. Heart failure usually ensues insidiously.

- Atrial standstill is described as **temporary** atrial standstill when it occurs as a consequence of a reversible condition. This maybe due to hyperkalaemia which can be secondary to Addison's disease, diabetic ketoacidosis and oliguric renal failure. Iatrogenic causes include excessive potassium infu-sion, transfusion of stored blood and potassium sparing diuretics. Digitalis toxicity is also a possible cause which can be established from the history and measurement of serum levels. The clinical signs are similar to persistent atrial standstill, with the addition of the signs related to the primary condition.

- Atrial standstill can occur in association with a 'dying' heart and is termed **terminal atrial standstill**.

Heart block

This is the failure of the depolarisation wave to conduct normally through the AV node, the correct term is therefore AV block. AV block may be partial (first or second degree block) or complete (third degree block).

First degree AV block

First degree AV block occurs when there is a delay in conduction through the AV node and there is usually a sinus rhythm.

ECG characteristics

The P wave and QRS complexes are normal in configuration, but the PR interval is prolonged (Fig. 10.4).

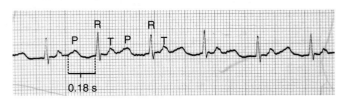

Figure 10.4 ECG from a cat showing a prolonged P–R interval, i.e. first degree AV (heart) block (50 mm/s and 1 cm/mV).

Clinical significance

First degree block does not, in itself, cause any clinical problems. It may occur normally in animals with a slow heart rate or in ageing animals due to degenerative changes in the AV node. The most common cause is probably due to digitalis toxicity or other drugs such as propranolol and procainamide. It may occur when there is an abnormal potassium level. Treatment should be aimed at correcting the underlying cause.

Second degree AV block

Second degree AV block occurs when conduction intermittently fails to pass through the AV node, i.e. there is atrial depolarisation which is not followed by ventricular depolarisation.

ECG characteristics

The P wave is normal, but there is either an occasional or frequent failure (depending on severity) of conduction through the AV node resulting in the absence of a QRS complex (Figs 9.11 and 10.5).

Second degree AV block can be classified further. When the P–R interval increases prior to the block it is termed **Mobitz type I** (also known as **Wenckebach's phenomenon**). But when the P–R interval remains constant prior to the block, this is termed **Mobitz type II** and the frequency of the block is usually constant, i.e. 2:1, 3:1 and so on.

Clinical significance

Mobitz type II

Advanced cases of second degree AV block may present with weakness, lethargy or syncope, it depends on the severity in the heart block and the consequent reduction in cardiac output. Auscultation reveals an intermittent pause in the cardiac rhythm. Second degree AV block that is severe or advanced (meaning the block occurs frequently) is usually Mobitz type

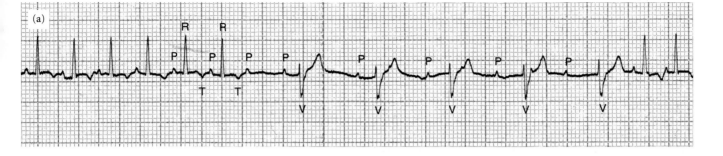

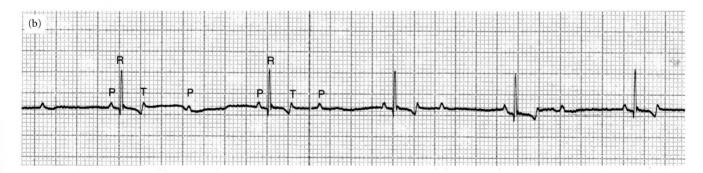

Figure 10.5 (a) ECG from a cat showing intermittently non-conducted P waves, i.e. second degree AV (heart) block, with ventricular escapes (labelled V) (25 mm/s and 1 cm/mV). (b) ECG from a 9-year-old Labrador with second degree AV block (25 mm/s and 0.5 cm/mV).

II. It is this type which may progress to complete AV block. It has been reported in older dogs with AV nodal fibrosis and hereditary stenosis of the bundle of His in the pug, however many cases are idiopathic. It may also occur with digitalis toxicity or other drugs, e.g. xylazine, detomodine, atropine and quinidine, or with a potassium imbalance. The author is also aware of some anecdotal reports of heart block in hypothyroid dogs.

Mobitz type I

Second degree AV block (Mobitz type I) is sometimes seen in normal dogs with sinus arrhythmia, particularly brachycephalic breeds.

Complete (third degree) AV block

Complete AV block occurs when there is a persistent failure of the depolarisation wave to be conducted through the AV node. A second pacemaker below the AV node (i.e. the block) discharges to control the ventricles. This second pacemaker may arise from:

- lower AV node or bundle branches producing a normal QRS (i.e. junctional escape complex) at approximately 60–70 per min
- Purkinje cells producing an abnormal QRS–T complex (i.e. ventricular escape complex) at approximately 30–40 per min.

ECG characteristics

On the ECG, P waves can be seen at a regular and fast rate but the QRS–T complexes are at a much slower rate, and usually fairly regular. The P waves and QRS complexes occur independently of the other (Fig. 10.6). This is best demonstrated by plotting out each P wave and each QRS complex on a piece of paper (Fig. 7.1).

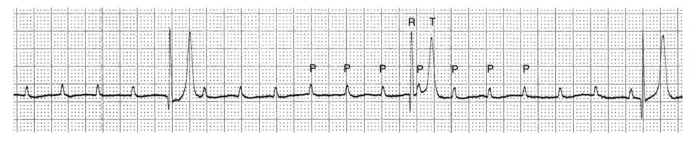

Figure 10.6 (a) ECG from an 8-year-old Labrador with third degree AV block (complete heart block) with a ventricular escape rhythm of 45/min (50 mm/s and 1 cm/mV).

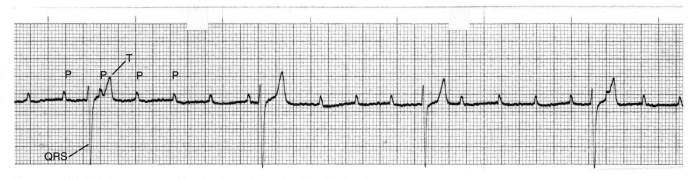

Figure 10.6 (b) ECG from a 10-year-old Collie dog with complete heart block with a slow ventricular escape rhythm at 30/min (25 mm/s and 1 cm/mV).

Clinical significance

The clinical signs may include weakness, lethargy, syncope or sudden death, depending on how slow the ventricular rate is, and the subsequent reduction in cardiac output. A very slow ventricular escape rhythm is usually associated with more marked clinical signs, with the possibility of sudden death. It is common in chronic cases, with a slow ventricular response rate, to find a generalised cardiomegaly with or without evidence of congestive heart failure on thoracic radiography. On auscultation a characteristic finding is a very regular and steady, but slow heart beat together with the palpation of a hyperdynamic femoral pulse. In some cases the more rapid atrial contraction sounds may be faintly audible. Complete AV block can be associated with cardiomyopathy, cardiac

neoplasia, digitalis toxicity, AV node fibrosis, endocarditis, electrolyte imbalance and Lyme disease.

Intraventricular conduction defects

The bundle of His divides into left and right bundle branches, supplying the left and right ventricles respectively (see page 5). The left bundle branch further divides into anterior and posterior fascicles. A block in conduction of the electrical impulse (similar to heart block described above) may occur in one or more of these conduction tissues, and in a number of combinations. The most commonly seen conduction defects seen in dogs and cats are:

- right bundle branch block (RBBB)
- left bundle branch block (LBBB)
- left anterior fascicular block (LAFB).

These result in abnormal depolarisation patterns as there will be a delay in depolarisation of the part of the ventricles supplied by the affected conduction tissue.

Right bundle branch block

Right bundle branch block (RBBB) occurs due to failure/delay of impulse conduction through the RBB. Depolarisation of the left ventricle occurs normally, but depolarisation of the right ventricular mass occurs through the myocardial cell tissue resulting in a very prolonged complex.

ECG characteristics

The QRS duration is prolonged (>0.07 seconds). The QRS complex has deep and usually slurred S waves in leads I, II, III and aVF and is positive in aVR and aVL. The MEA is to the right (Fig. 10.7a). Note that RBBB needs to be differentiated from a right ventricular enlargement pattern.

An animal with atrial fibrillation can concurrently have bundle branch block (Fig. 10.7b), this is often a more challenging ECG interpretation!

(a)

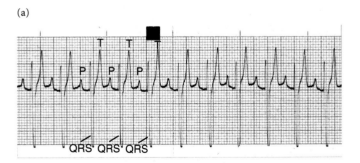

(b)

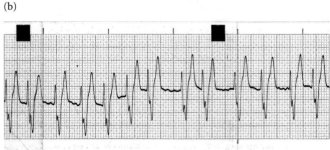

Figure 10.7 (a) ECG (lead II) from a 10-year-old mixed breed dog with a normal sinus rhythm at 140/min, but conducted with aberrancy through the ventricles due to right bundle branch block. This was an incidental finding. Note the abnormal morphology of the QRS complexes, with deep (negative) Q waves and prolonged QRS duration. There is a P for every QRS, indicating the sinus origin of the depolarisation (25 mm/s and 1 cm/mV). (b) ECG (lead II) from dog with atrial fibrillation (note the irregular R–R intervals and the fibrillation waves) and right bundle branch block (deep S waves and prolonged QRS durations) (25 mm/s and 1 cm/mV).

Clinical significance

The right bundle branch (RBBB) is long and slender, thus vulnerable to damage. RBBB is not uncommon in normal healthy dogs but can be associated with congenital or acquired heart disease, cardiac neoplasia and trauma. RBBB, in itself, does not cause any significant haemodynamic problems, however, if damage to the left bundle branch were also to occur it would lead to complete heart block.

Left bundle branch block

Left bundle branch block (LBBB) occurs due to failure of conduction through the LBB. Depolarisation of the right ventricle occurs normally and depolarisation of the left ventricle is delayed and occurs through the myocardial cell tissue resulting in a very prolonged complex.

ECG characteristics

The QRS duration is very prolonged (>0.07 seconds). There are positive complexes in leads I, II, III and aVF and negative in aVR and aVL (Fig. 10.8). LBBB needs to be differentiated from a left ventricular enlargement pattern.

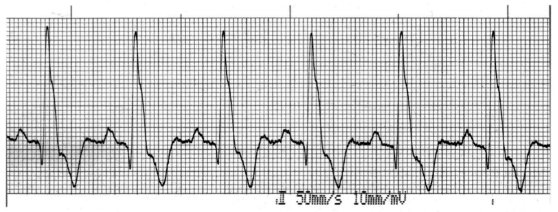

Figure 10.8 ECG from a dog with a normal sinus rhythm conducted through the ventricles with aberrancy due to left bundle branch block. Note the abnormal morphology of the QRS complexes, yet related to the P waves, i.e. there is a P for every QRS, indicating the sinus origin of the depolarisations (50 mm/s and 1 cm/mV).

Clinical significance

The left bundle branch is thick and therefore a larger lesion is required to produce conduction block. LBBB is therefore rare in normal healthy animals and when it does occur is often associated with pathology: congenital (e.g. subaortic stenosis) or acquired heart disease (e.g. hypertrophic or dilated cardiomyopathy), myocardial ischaemia, cardiac neoplasia or trauma. In itself, it does not cause any significant haemodynamic problems.

Left anterior fascicular block

Left anterior fascicular block (LAFB) occurs due to failure of conduction through the anterior fascicle of the LBB. It is not an uncommon finding in cats but is rare in the dog.

ECG characteristics

The QRS complex is normal in duration but there are tall R waves in leads I and aVL, deep S waves (>R wave) in leads II, III and aVF. The MEA is markedly to the left; approx. −60° in the cat (Fig. 10.9a).

A cat with atrial fibrillation can also concurrently have fascicular block (Fig. 10.9b).

Clinical significance

It is often considered a relatively specific indicator of hypertrophic cardiomyopathy in the cat (although it can be seen with many heart diseases in cats). It can be associated with hypertrophic or restrictive cardiomyopathy, electrolyte imbalance such as hyperkalaemia.

Ventricular pre-excitation

This occurs when the impulse from the SA node bypasses the AV node through an accessory conduction pathway to the ventricles and therefore depolarises the ventricles prematurely. The impulse conducted through the accessory pathway stimulates a portion of the ventricles with the rest of the ventricles being activated in the normal sequence through the AV node. There are believed to be three accessory pathways: bundles of Kent, James fibres and Mahaim fibres.

The **Wolff–Parkinson–White** (WPW) syndrome consists of ventricular pre-excitation with episodes of paroxysmal supraventricular tachycardia.

The heart rhythm (except with WPW syndrome) is unaffected and is usually regular.

ECG characteristics

The electrocardiographic characteristics are within the P–QRS–T complex itself. There is a short PR interval, a slur or notch (delta wave) in the upstroke of the R wave and a slight prolongation of the QRS complex. In WPW syndrome the supraventricular tachycardia is often in excess of 300 per min.

(a)

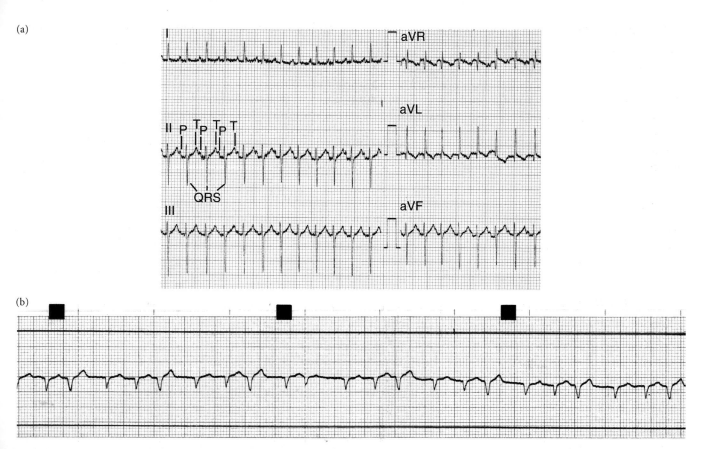

(b)

Figure 10.9 (a) ECG from a cat with taurine responsive dilated cardiomyopathy. There is a normal sinus rhythm but aberrant ventricular conduction due to anterior fascicular block (see text) (25 mm/s and 1 cm/mV). (b) ECG from a cat with atrial fibrillation and anterior fascicular block.

Clinical significance

Ventricular pre-excitation itself is not haemodynamically significant, however, WPW syndrome may cause weakness or syncope, as the very rapid tachycardia is associated with marked reduction in cardiac output. Pre-excitation may be present as a congenital lesion with or without organic heart disease.

Further reading

As a general reference guide the follow text is recommended:

Tilley (1992) *Essentials of canine and feline electrocardiography: Interpretation and treatment*, 3rd edition. Lea & Febiger.

For practising reading ECGs, which is strongly recommended:

Tilley (1992) *Self assessment: Small animal arrhythmias*. Lea & Febiger.

An audiotape and workbook:

Smith & Tilley (1992) *Rapid interpretation of heart sounds, murmurs, and arrhythmias*. Lea & Febiger.

Books on veterinary cardiology.

Martin & Corcoran (1997) *Cardiorespiratory diseases of the dog and cat*. Blackwell Science.

Darke, Bonagura & Kelly (1996) *Color atlas of veterinary cardiology*. Mosby-Wolfe.

Fox (1999) *Canine and feline cardiology*. WB Saunders.

Kittleson & Kienle (1998) *Small animal cardiovascular medicine*. Mosby.

Index